THE TRIATHLETE'S TRAINING DIARY

2nd EDITION

THE TRIATHLETE'S TRAINING DIARY

2nd EDITION

YOUR ULTIMATE TOOL FOR FASTER, STRONGER RACING

JOE FRIEL

VELO.
press

▼velopress®

an imprint of Ulysses Press
PO Box 3440
Berkeley, CA 94703
www.velopress.com

ISBN: 978-1-64604-659-1
Library of Congress Control Number: 2023945736

Printed in the United States
10 9 8 7 6 5 4 3 2 1

Front and back cover photos by Michael Rauschendorfer; inside cover photo by
Paul Phillips/Competitive Image; and photo on page 29 by Nils Nilsen

CONTENTS

Any coach will tell you that a carefully maintained training record is a great tool for faster, stronger racing. Some triathletes and duathletes are good at keeping a training diary, but others fail to take the time. Without a diary you're forced to rely on memory, which all too often recalls only exaggerated versions of what happened months, weeks, or even days before.

There are several other good reasons to keep a diary. It can serve as a positive reinforcement and boost confidence before particularly challenging races. By looking back to workouts or other races that loomed large but were mastered, you can feel assured that you have what it takes. A diary also reveals whether your fitness is improving by comparing recent measures such as time trials, interval results, or even resting heart rates against similar standards a year or more ago, when you were in great shape. In the same way, you can thumb back through a diary to discover what has and hasn't worked before. This could be a peaking procedure prior to an especially good race, a way of dealing with an injury that once proved successful, or a pacing strategy that worked well.

Perhaps the main argument for using a diary is in the prevention of overtraining—a necessity for nearly every serious athlete. More on this later.

WHAT IS A TRAINING DIARY?

Record-keeping works best in accomplishing these objectives if it's in the form of both a daily log and journal. Technically, a log is a record of basic data, usually numbers, that relate to progress (distance, time, heart rate, etc.), while a journal is a record of your thoughts and experiences. Log information is objective, while the journal portion is subjective. Both are important. By combining the two into a diary, the information you collect covers a broader spectrum of needs.

You may decide not to use all of the spaces provided in this diary—that's okay. Whatever you write down, make it only what's important and useful to you. Everything else just gets in the way when trying to analyze your training.

THE "O" WORD

The diary is most commonly used to avoid overtraining. When it seems that training isn't going well, and you aren't quite sure why, looking back through diary notes for the last few weeks may reveal a cause. Look for phrases used repeatedly such as "feel tired" or "no snap today" or "sluggish." These are sure signs that you're doing too much—overreaching. Also check the numbers for trends and patterns. You may find that every third day or so, sleep quality is poor and fatigue is high. Such a pattern is telling you to allow more recovery time between the hard workouts. Another possible sign of doing too much is when heart rate data and workout ratings don't agree. For example, your heart rate is low, but the effort seems high. Such a review of the training diary helps you decide if it's time to take a long break or to just cut back for a couple of days.

JUST SAY NO TO COMPULSION

Keeping a diary is helpful for making progress in triathlon and duathlon, but don't let it become a handicap to your training and racing. Athletes who believe they must achieve and record certain numbers in their training diary each week often lose focus of what swimming, biking, and running are all about—having fun! This diary is merely a tool to help you achieve your fitness goals and record what you accomplish this year. Using a training diary as described here won't guarantee your success in races. It will, however, increase the likelihood.

HOW TO PLAN YOUR SEASON

Multisport athletes are goal-driven people. Show me a triathlete or duathlete who has no desire to swim, bike, and run stronger and faster, and I'll show you an athlete who will not be in the sport for long. Success is not possible in multisport without high motivation. Triathlon and duathlon are just too grueling to do in an indifferent manner. Every athlete wants to improve, but a passion to excel is nothing without a passion to prepare to excel.

Preparation is where many athletes fail. Most are willing to put in endless hours on the road or in the pool but are less zealous when it comes to planning. That's a shame, because planning is the first step in achieving any goal in life, including for those accomplished in endurance sports. A goal without a plan is just a wish.

Most athletes could achieve their goals by making only one small change: writing down a plan for how to train throughout the year. Just as with a diary, training plans may comprise the most minute particulars or provide just a rough outline. Regardless of the detail, better racing will result from deciding in advance what you'll do in training and when.

The Annual Training Plan is a tool that will help you incorporate periodization into your training. Periodization is a way of training in which fitness is built from the most basic to the more complex aspects in stages or periods. The purpose of periodization is fast racing when it counts.

The following step-by-step description guides you through each part of the Annual Training Plan that follows. It may take you 30 minutes or so to design your personal plan, but it's time well invested. It's best to write only in pencil, as things are likely to change during the season. You can see a sample completed plan on pages 8–9.

STEP 1: SET YOUR SEASON GOALS

What are three major racing accomplishments you'd like to achieve this year? Write them down on the Annual Training Plan (see page 19). Keep it to three or fewer, as having more is likely to complicate your training and racing.

Goals are best if they're realistic, specific, measurable, and performance-oriented. For example:

Break 2:30 for an international distance race by August 1.

Also write your goals on the jacket flap so that you'll see them every time you open your diary. Goals are most effective when they're written down and reviewed frequently.

STEP 2: IDENTIFY YOUR TRAINING OBJECTIVES

Training objectives are the aspects of fitness or the workout performances needed to achieve your season goals. Just as with the goals, objectives are best if they are realistic, specific, measurable, and performance-oriented. Write these objectives on the jacket flap so you'll see them often. An example of a training objective that might support the above example of a season goal is:

Run a 10K race in less than 45 minutes by July 15.

STEP 3: ESTABLISH YOUR ANNUAL HOURS

How many hours did you train last year? Are you capable of doing more, or do you need to cut back this year due to time constraints? Would you like to race more competitively this year, or is this a year just to maintain your race level?

The answers to these questions will help you decide how many hours to train in the coming year. There is a relationship between how many hours or miles you covered in a year and how you race. If you're unsure of your hours from last year due to poor record-keeping, now is a good time to start rectifying that problem.

Here are suggested annual hours by race distance. These are not absolutes; in other words, you don't have to train at these hours to race competitively or even complete these race distances. Some athletes do more and still race poorly. Others do less and win frequently.

race distance	annual hours
Ironman®	600–1,200
Half-Ironman	500–700
Olympic	400–600
Sprint	300–500
Juniors	200–350

STEP 4: FILL IN THE CALENDAR

In the column titled "Mon." write in the dates of each Monday in the year. For example, if the first Monday in January is January 5, write "1/5."

STEP 5: PLAN YOUR YEAR OF RACING

List all of the races you may do this year in the "races" column, placing them in the proper weeks according to their dates. If unsure about a particular race, list it.

STEP 6: PRIORITIZE YOUR RACES

Give a priority ranking (in the column labeled "pri.") to each of the races using the following guidelines:

A-Priority Races. These are the most important races—the ones that will determine success in the coming season. They are closely related to the Season Goals on the previous page. You will peak and taper for each of these races. Limit these to no more than three or four A races in a year. Two in the same week counts as one A race. Trying to peak more times than this prevents you from coming into top form since tapering actually reduces some aspects of fitness, and there may not be enough time between them to regain lost fitness.

B-Priority Races. These aren't as important as the A races, so there isn't any peaking and tapering. Two to four days of rest, however, precede each of them. Assign a B priority to up to eight races, again counting two in the same week as one.

C-Priority Races. These least important races are ones that you may not even do. You can decide at the last minute. You'll "train through them," meaning they are treated the same as hard workouts. They are best used as tune-up races before A- and B-priority races. They also make good workouts and build experience in novices. There is no limit on the number of C races, but they can interfere with training, so choose them conservatively. Frequent racing without a break is a common cause of burnout and overtraining.

STEP 7: IDENTIFY YOUR TRAINING PERIODS

This step is where the periodization begins. You will now divide the season into periods starting with your A races. A clumping of A-priority races is called a "race" period and may last as long as 6 weeks or as short as 1. The week or two before each race period, write in "peak." Preceding each of these peaks is a 6- to 10-week "build" period. The first build period of the year is preceded by an 8- to 12-week "base" period and before that a 3- to 4-week "prep" period. It's a good idea to plan for some rest after each of the race periods by plugging in a 3-day to 6-week "transition." Use a short transition early in the season and a longer one later in the season following A-priority races.

The suggested characteristics of each of these periods are as follows:

Prep. General adaptation to training with weights; crosstraining; and swim, bike, and run drills.

Base. Gradually establish the basic fitness elements of endurance, hill strength for running and biking, and leg and arm speed. Begin muscular endurance with training near lactate threshold.

Build. Develop greater race-specific fitness with intervals and tempo workouts while refining muscular endurance and hill strength. Maintain endurance and leg and arm speed. Work especially on improving personal racing limiters and achieving Training Objectives.

Peak. Reduce volume and allow for more recovery days between hard workouts that simulate racing, such as bricks, and refine needed skills. These mini-race simulations are done every third or fourth day in this period.

Race. A period of focused racing with greatly reduced training.

Transition. An extended period of rest and recovery.

You can use the blank monthly calendars (pages 22–25) to keep track of what months your different training periods will fall in. These calendars are also useful to help you schedule testing and to decide what days of the week are best to do particular workouts. Filling in these calendars will help you see your progression of weekly hours from month to month as well as your progression of races for the entire year. The calendars may also serve as reminders to plan your training around events in your work or personal life.

STEP 8: FILL IN YOUR WEEKLY HOURS

Write in the approximate number of hours you will train each week, including weights and crosstraining, based on the Weekly Training Hours table (see pages 26–27). The actual hours you work out each week will vary from this based on many circumstances such as weather or other complications. This is a guideline only. Feel free to change it to meet your exact needs.

Divide hours between the three sports in a way that reflects the nature of the event for which you're preparing, and your racing limiters. For example, most triathlons are lopsided in favor of the bike leg, while the swim is relatively short. Weekly bike and swim training times may reflect this; however, if swimming is a weak sport for you and biking is stronger, favoring the swim with a disproportionately high number of hours is often a wise decision. Most duathlons are fairly well balanced as far as duration of the combined race legs, but a weakness in one might cause you to favor it.

STEP 9: TARGET YOUR MOST IMPORTANT WORKOUTS

Each week check the key workout types for each sport, following the period guidelines offered in Step 7. Key workouts are described in the following terms. (For more details of each of these types of workouts, see *The Triathlete's Training Bible*.)

Endurance. These workouts emphasize the athlete's ability to delay the onset of fatigue and reduce its effects. This may include longer, low-intensity work.

Muscular Force. These workouts improve ability to overcome resistance— for example, swimming in rough water or running or biking on hills or in the wind.

Speed Skills. These are workouts that train an athlete to move effectively in each sport, usually emphasizing form and technique.

Muscular Endurance. These are workouts that train muscles to maintain a relatively high force load for a prolonged period of time by combining force and endurance training.

Anaerobic Endurance. These workouts emphasize the athlete's ability to resist fatigue at a very high level of effort with high arm or leg turnover. This type of training is best introduced later in the season.

Sprint Power. This training develops the athlete's ability to apply maximum force quickly. This type of training usually involves short, all-out efforts and is best done early in a training session before the body is fatigued.

Testing. Performed on recovery weeks, testing is a good way to measure your progress throughout a season.

For an example of a completed plan, see pages 8–9.

HOW TO USE THIS DIARY

A training diary is only as useful as you make it. If you record little or write in it inconsistently, a diary has little value. On the other hand, recording lots of needless data that you never look at again not only wastes time but also makes it harder to analyze later. The key is to write down immediately following every workout what was important, and nothing more. The longer you wait, the greater the possibility you'll forget something or those feelings will fade.

To ensure that it's used, keep this diary in a place that you go after every workout, perhaps where you store your workout gear. That way you see it and are more likely to

ANNUAL HOURS — 500 hours

week	Mon.	races	pri.	period	vol.	WEIGHTS	swim							bike							run						
							AEROBIC ENDURANCE	MUSCULAR FORCE	SPEED SKILLS	MUSCULAR ENDURANCE	ANAEROBIC ENDURANCE	SPRINT POWER	TESTING	AEROBIC ENDURANCE	MUSCULAR FORCE	SPEED SKILLS	MUSCULAR ENDURANCE	ANAEROBIC ENDURANCE	SPRINT POWER	TESTING	AEROBIC ENDURANCE	MUSCULAR FORCE	SPEED SKILLS	MUSCULAR ENDURANCE	ANAEROBIC ENDURANCE	SPRINT POWER	TESTING
01	11/21			prep	8.5	AA	X		X					X	X						X		X				
02	11/28			↓	8.5	AA	X		X				X	X	X					X	X		X				X
03	12/5			base	10.0	MT	X		X					X	X						X		X				
04	12/12				12.0	MT	X		X					X	X						X		X				
05	12/19				13.5	MS	X		X					X	X						X		X				
06	12/26			↓	7.0	MS	X		X				X	X	X					X	X		X				X
07	1/2			base 2	10.5	MS	X		X	X				X	X						X		X	X			
08	1/9				12.5	MS	X		X	X				X	X						X		X	X			
09	1/16				19.0	SM	X	X	X	X				X	X	X	X				X	X	X	X			
10	1/23			↓	7.0	SM	X		X				X	X	X					X	X		X				X
11	1/30			base 3	11.0	SM	X	X	X	X	X			X	X	X	X	X			X	X	X	X	X		
12	2/6				13.5	SM	X	X	X	X	X			X	X	X	X	X			X	X	X	X	X		
13	2/13	(Tri camp)			15.0	SM	X	X	X	X	X			X	X	X	X	X			X	X	X	X	X		
14	2/20	Sprint Tri Race	C	↓	7.0	SM	X		X				X	X	X					X	X		X				X
15	2/27			build 1	12.5	SM	X	X	X	X	X			X	X	X	X	X			X	X	X	X	X		
16	3/6				12.5	SM	X	X	X	X	X			X	X	X	X	X			X	X	X	X	X		
17	3/13				12.5	SM	X	X	X	X	X			X	X	X	X	X			X	X	X	X	X		
18	3/20	Olympic Tri Race	B	↓	7.0	SM	X		X				X	X	X					X	X		X				X
19	3/27			build 2	13.0	SM	X	X	X	X	X			X	X	X	X	X			X	X	X	X	X		
20	4/3				12.0	SM	X	X	X	X	X			X	X	X	X	X			X	X	X	X	X		
21	4/10				12.0	SM	X	X	X	X	X			X	X	X	X	X			X	X	X	X	X		
22	4/17	10K Run Race	B	↓	7.0	SM	X		X				X	X	X					X	X		X				X
23	4/24			peak	10.5	SM				X							X							X			
24	5/1			↓	8.5	SM				X							X							X			
25	5/8	Gulf Coast HIM	A	race	7.0	SM				X							X							X			
26	5/15			trans.	—																						

week	Mon.	races	pri.	period	vol.	WEIGHTS	swim AER.END.	swim MUSC.FORCE	swim SPEED SKILLS	swim MUSC.END.	swim ANAER.END.	swim SPRINT PWR	swim TESTING	bike AER.END.	bike MUSC.FORCE	bike SPEED SKILLS	bike MUSC.END.	bike ANAER.END.	bike SPRINT PWR	bike TESTING	run AER.END.	run MUSC.FORCE	run SPEED SKILLS	run MUSC.END.	run ANAER.END.	run SPRINT PWR	run TESTING
27	5/22			base 3	11.0	MS	X	X	X	X				X	X	X	X				X	X	X	X			
28	5/29				13.5	MS	X	X	X	X				X	X	X	X				X	X	X	X			
29	6/25			↓	7.0	MS	X		X					X	X		X				X		X				X
30	6/12			base 3	13.5	SM	X	X	X	X	X			X	X	X	X	X			X	X	X	X	X		
31	6/19				15.0	SM	X	X	X	X	X			X	X	X	X	X			X	X	X	X	X		
32	6/26			↓	7.0	SM	X		X					X	X		X				X		X				X
33	7/3			base 3	13.5	SM	X	X	X	X	X			X	X	X	X	X			X	X	X	X	X		
34	7/10				15.0	SM	X	X	X	X	X			X	X	X	X	X			X	X	X	X	X		
35	7/17	Half Marathon	B	↓	7.0	SM	X		X					X	X		X				X		X				X
36	7/24			build 1	12.5	SM	X	X	X	X	X			X	X	X	X	X			X	X	X	X	X		
37	7/31				12.5	SM	X	X	X	X	X			X	X	X	X	X			X	X	X	X	X		
38	8/7	Olympic Tri Race	C		12.5	SM	X	X	X	X	X			X	X	X	X	X			X	X	X	X	X		
39	8/14			↓	7.0	SM	X		X					X	X		X				X		X				X
40	8/21			build 2	12.0	SM	X	X	X	X	X			X	X	X	X	X			X	X	X	X	X		
41	8/28				12.0	SM	X	X	X	X	X			X	X	X	X	X			X	X	X	X	X		
42	9/4				12.0	SM	X	X	X	X	X			X	X	X	X	X			X	X	X	X	X		
43	9/11	Olympic Tri Race	B	↓	7.0	SM	X		X					X	X		X				X		X				X
44	9/18			peak	10.5	SM				X							X							X			
45	9/25			↓	8.5	SM				X							X							X			
46	10/2	Silverman 70.3	A	race	7.0	SM				X							X							X			
47	10/9			trans.	—																						
48	10/16				—																						
49	10/23				—																						
50	10/30				—																						
51	11/6																										
52	11/3																										

write in it right away. Your log is a constant reminder of your goals and progress. Filling it out after every workout will help to keep you on track throughout the season.

The text that follows describes the various parts of the diary pages that make up most of this book. You may decide not to use some parts, or you may want to modify the information you record in other parts from what is suggested here. The most important point is that you keep an accurate record of training and racing for future reference. The bold headings listed here can be found on each diary page.

WEEK BEGINNING

At the start of each week indicate Monday's date. These correspond with the "Mon." column of the Annual Training Plan.

week beginning:	_March 5_
period: _build 1_	planned hours: _15:00_

PERIOD

Indicate what training period this week falls into: prep, base, build, peak, race, or transition. This is found in the "period" column on the Annual Training Plan. Knowing which period you are in helps you decide what workouts to do throughout the week (see *The Triathlete's Training Bible* for details).

PLANNED HOURS

The approximate number of hours you plan to train this week is recorded here based on what you wrote on the Annual Training Plan in the "hours" column. This is a rough guideline only. You may decide to change this a little one way or the other. The idea, however, is to remain consistent with your plan so that a high-volume week remains much the same, as does a low-volume recovery week. On the other hand, if you aren't feeling right late in the week, it's better to cut back than to risk overtraining or illness. When in doubt, cut it out.

WEEK GOALS

At the start of each week, write in three goals you want to accomplish that will help achieve your training objectives on the Annual Training Plan. For example, if one of your training objectives is "Run a 10K race in less than 45 minutes by July 15," then at some point in the season, after building the necessary fitness, this becomes a weekly goal. Prior to that, other weekly goals will build up to this. For example, "Run 4 × 1 mile at 7:30 pace with 30-second recoveries." Check off each of your goals as you achieve them.

---

week goals: ✓ *Run 4 x 1 mile at 7:30 pace with 30-second recoveries*
✓ *Ride 6 x 1-mile hill repeats in various gears – easy to hard*
✓ *Conduct a 1,500-meter time trial*

MONDAY_____

Write in Monday's date (also write in dates for the other days of the week).

MONDAY _____ 3 / 13 / 17 _____
2 sleep 4 fatigue 1 stress 2 soreness
resting heart rate_____ +5 _____ weight _____ 150 _____

VITAL SIGNS (SLEEP, FATIGUE, STRESS, SORENESS)

The purpose of this part of the diary is to help you listen to your body. Every day it gives you clues about what condition it is in. By closely monitoring some of the signals it sends out, you can head off overtraining, burnout, injury, and illness.

The first thing you should do every morning is rate your perceptions of the previous night's sleep, your fatigue level, psychological stress, and soreness. Use a scale of 1 to 7 with 1 being the best, most favorable rating, and 7 the worst, most unfavorable rating. Write the appropriate number in the space preceding each signal.

Resting heart rate should be taken while you are still in bed and recorded as beats per minute (bmp) above (+) or below (−) normal, based on a one-week average found when you were well rested. While a low resting heart rate is usually a good sign for fitness, it is not always so. Some scientific studies have found obviously overtrained athletes with low resting heart rates.

A rating of 4 or greater on any of these vital signs should be considered as a warning that something isn't right. The more warnings, the more cautiously and conservatively you should train on that day.

Also record your body weight right after getting out of bed. Fluctuations in weight could indicate that your diet is out of harmony with your needs. It could also be due to low hydration levels, emotional stress, or high training workloads. Consider a two-pound change in two days as a sign that something is wrong.

WORKOUTS 1 AND 2

Circle S (swim), B (bike), or R (run) to indicate the mode of the workout planned for that day. If it is something other than swimming, biking, or running, circle O (other) and write in what it is. This could be strength training, a yoga class, or any other cross-training you may do.

PLANNED WORKOUT

At the start of the week, briefly summarize what you'll do in training each day and the intended duration of each workout. This will only take 5 to 10 minutes and is time well spent when you consider how much time you put into daily training. The columns on the right side of your Annual Training Plan labeled "swim," "bike," and "run" will help with this task. (The details of each of these types of workouts are found in *The Triathlete's Training Bible*.)

Notice that there is only room for two workouts per day. Few multisport athletes, mostly pros, need to train more than twice a day. For nearly everyone else, a regular diet of three-a-day workouts is a good way to wind up overtrained.

You may even develop a code for specific workouts that you do frequently. And, for easier access, write these codes on the inside of the diary's cover flap. In this part, also write in the planned duration of the workout in time or distance. These daily duration totals should be approximately equal to the "hours" column for that week on the Annual Training Plan.

> **WORKOUT 1** S (B) R O _____
> planned workout _2 hours with 4 x 10-_
> _minute zone 4 (3-min. recoveries)_
> route _Nelson loop_

WORKOUT DETAILS

As soon as you finish the workout, record the details—route, distance, time, average heart rate, etc. Most multisport athletes have common bike and run routes with short names. You may want to note these in the "Routes and Best Times" section in the back of the diary (page 262). Also write in the distance covered in the workout and the time, either elapsed workout time or time of day. Record your average heart rate for the workout.

AVERAGE HEART RATE AND POWER

Average heart rate (avg. HR) and average power (avg. power) are good indicators of how intense your workout was. Also, by comparing the two, you can get an excellent indicator of how your fitness is progressing. Divide your average power by your average heart rate to get a sense of how hard you are working to produce a certain level of power. Over time, this number will increase as your fitness improves.

ZONE 1_____ 2_____ 3_____ 4_____ 5_____

Summarize the heart rate intensity of the workout in these spaces by indicating how many minutes were spent in each zone. If your monitor has memory, you can easily indicate three zones ("above," "in," and "below" in heart rate monitor language). This is important information that will indicate whether you're getting enough appropriate-intensity training early in the season, and whether the weekly volume in the race-specific zones is adequate later in the season when a race period approaches. When you fill out this section following a race, it will give you a better insight as to the intensities necessary to race and thus to train.

> dist. _42_ time _2:22_ avg. HR ___136___
> zone 1 _40_ 2 _67_ 3 _304_ _55_ 5 ___0___

NOTES

This is the journal part of the diary. Record comments about your workout such as whom you trained with, how you felt, interval heart rates and times, pace, power, soreness, noticed improvements, results of self-tests, or outside factors such as work that left you tired. Later, as you go back over the diary trying to figure why you raced as you did, these comments will give life to the workout details logged earlier.

It's also a good idea to record any changes made to your equipment in this part, such as new running shoes, a new bike seat position, or new pedals. A few days or weeks later some problem such as knee pain may appear, and knowing what changes were made and when the changes were made helps in the detective work. You can also note such bike setup changes on the bike measurement charts near the back of the diary (see pages 260–261).

NUTRITION

Other than high-quality workouts and rest, nothing has as great an impact on your training and race performance as what you eat and when you eat it. Use this space to record any number of nutrition details for the day such as calories consumed; carbo-hydrate, fat, and protein intake; supplements used; dietary changes; your nutrition "grade" for the day; or anything else you feel is important.

WEEKLY SUMMARY

Summarize the week by totaling weekly swim, bike, and run times and distances. There is also space to total time and distance for the Year to Date (YTD). This will come in handy at the end of the season when you start planning for next year. Keeping it tallied weekly is easier than going back and adding up a year of entries. "Strength" tracks time in the weight room. "Other" is for crosstraining activities such as cross-country skiing. Write in which activity was done and the totals.

WEEKLY SUMMARY

	time	distance	YTD time	YTD distance
swim	3:15	9000m	65:00	190.143 mi
bike	4:00	80 mi	80:00	1,400 mi
run	3:00	22.5 mi	62:00	380 mi
strength	1:00		23:00	
other XC ski	3:00	20 mi	10:00	60 mi
total	14:15		240:00	
notes	A bit sore — back off next week.			

In the "Notes" section briefly summarize how the week went. Describe any soreness encountered, no matter how slight, in case it recurs or becomes worse. Knowing when it started may help determine a cause. Brief, to-the-point comments are more likely to help you later than overly detailed discussions. This is also a good place to give yourself a pat on the back—or a kick in the pants—depending on how you did this week.

RACE _Boulder Peak_   _7 / 9 / 17_   distance _Oly_

location _Boulder, CO_   time _2:16:24_ placement overall _4_   AG _2_

	time	distance	pace	place
swim	23:16	1500 m	1:33/100 m	45
bike	1:06:13	40K	22:17 mph	31
run	45:06	10K	7:16/mi	36
transition 1		1:06		
transition 2		0:43		

nutrition pre-race _applesauce with protein powder_

nutrition during race _sports drink, gel_

avg. heart rate _155_ max heart rate _163_ avg. power _205_

notes _Need to swim more consistently with masters. Felt strong on bike and ran well despite hot day. Did a good job of fueling._

OTHER DIARY USES

A training diary is the best place to store all sorts of basic information about your training, equipment, race results, and other personal details. At some time in the future—next month, next year, or three years from now—something will come up that you need to remember. How did I do in this race last time? How much volume did I do in my best year? How was my last bike set up? How much intense training did I do last spring? This section will provide the answers quickly.

The pages at the back offer ample room to keep track of many details and to customize them to fit your exact needs and interests. Here are some possibilities.

RACE RESULTS

Here (see page 242) you can summarize the important details of your races including race name, date, location, distance, finish time, overall placement, and age group (AG) placement. Record how you did for each part of the race. In the "Notes" section add a personal evaluation of your performance, including opportunities for improvement.

TEST RESULTS

Periodic fitness testing is a great way to know if your training is on track. You may have a gut feeling that you are in better shape now than a few weeks ago, but without some hard evidence there's no way to be sure. In this section (see page 248) you can record the results of your tests for future reference. Having test results from a period when you know you were in great shape serves as a standard to gauge the results of similar tests in the future.

TEST TYPE

There are two general categories of tests—field tests and lab tests. And within those two broad categories there are more-defined testing protocols. See *The Triathlete's Training Bible* for examples of field tests you may do, such as a Graded Exercise Test, Aerobic Time Trial, or 30-Minute Time Trial.

HEART RATE AND POWER AT ANAEROBIC THRESHOLD

Many of the tests you do can help you determine your anaerobic (lactate) threshold (AT). This is a critical physiological point that can be generally defined as the intensity level at which lactate accumulates in your bloodstream more quickly than it can be processed. The most common indicators used to identify your AT are heart rate and power. Whenever a test identifies either of these landmarks, record it here.

ZONES

Once you know your AT, you can set up training intensity zones for power and heart rate. Again, see *The Triathlete's Training Bible* for heart rate zones. For power, use these ranges:

Zone 1 less than 56% of AT power

Zone 2 56–75% of AT power

Zone 3 76–90% of AT power

Zone 4 91–100% of AT power

Zone 5a 101–105% of AT power

Zone 5b 106–120% of AT power

Zone 5c more than 120% of AT power

VO₂MAX AND BODY FAT

If your test identifies these metrics, record them here for future reference.

NOTES

Make notes on details that have an effect on test results such as equipment used, pre-test meals, warm-up, and equipment calibration. Also record the precise protocol used in the test.

TRAINING GRIDS

Training and fitness trends are more easily seen when information is graphed. The blank grids provided on pages 251–259 can be used to record the training data that are most important to you on a monthly and yearly basis. For example, you may choose to display weekly training hours or distances by sport; the longest weekly workout; the volume of weekly, race-specific intensity training (a good predictor of performance); or daily heart rates (waking, recovery, or post-workout).

Here's an idea that both combines the duration of a workout with its intensity and is easily graphed to reveal how hard you're actually training: Assign a "workload" value to each workout. One way of doing this is to multiply the number of minutes in a zone by the numeric name of the heart rate zone. For example, if you spent 10 minutes in zone 4 during a given training session, the workload is 40 (10 × 4) for that portion of the workout. The total workload for a session is the combined workloads for each of the five heart rate zones. While not a perfect system, this allows you to roughly determine what kind of stress is applied each day or week and to compare workouts between sports. Graphing cumulative workloads for each week on one of these grids, rather than merely recording miles, gives you a better idea of how your training is really going. Below is an example for one month of running workouts.

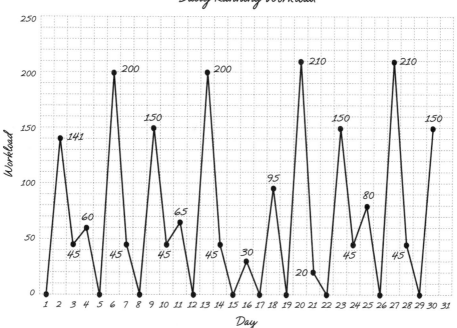

Daily Running Workload

BIKE MEASUREMENT CHARTS

Have you ever changed your saddle position and then tried to set it back to the original position only to find that it was never quite right again? Completing the diagrams on pages 260–261 with your exact measurements will resolve this once and for all. Doing so will also allow you to set up a new bike to your exact position without a lot of trial and error. Any time equipment is changed, having a position record can potentially save lots of time and frustration.

ROUTES AND BEST TIMES

If you're like most multisport athletes, you have established routes that you frequently run and ride. Sometimes at the end of a workout you realize that you went especially fast and you try to remember what your times were like on this same course before. Here is the place to note such times for later reference.

Another use for this section is as a record of self-tests. For example, pick out a flat 5- to 10-mile course with no stop streets and ride it at a given heart rate, say 9 to 11 beats below your lactate threshold heart rate, in a standard gear. If you've done a good job of controlling variables such as warm-up, rest, diet, and weather, decreasing times are a sign that fitness is improving. The same procedure is possible on the running track for 1 to 5 miles. This is called an "aerobic time trial."

Monthly, all-out time trials on a standard course or track also serve as good indicators of progress when done regularly, especially before the race season begins.

RACE-DAY CHECKLIST

Almost every athlete forgets something critical on race day, like shoes or a helmet, at least once a year. Sometimes your memory just isn't good enough to recall all of the many items you need. The night before a race, gather your gear together and check it off in pencil (see page 264). That reduces the race-day stress the next morning and allows your mind to relax and think about racing well instead of wondering whether or not you packed your sunglasses.

Whether you work with a coach or train independently, there is a lot to learn over the course of a year of swimming, biking, and running. I hope that you will use this diary to improve your performance in triathlon and get even more enjoyment from the sport in the years to come.

annual training plan

SEASON GOALS

1. _____

_____

_____

2. _____

_____

_____

3. _____

_____

_____

TRAINING OBJECTIVES

1. _____

_____

_____

2. _____

_____

_____

3. _____

_____

_____

4. _____

_____

_____

5. _____

_____

_____

ANNUAL HOURS _____

week	Mon.	races	pri.	period	vol.	WEIGHTS	swim							bike							run						
							AEROBIC ENDURANCE	MUSCULAR FORCE	SPEED SKILLS	MUSCULAR ENDURANCE	ANAEROBIC ENDURANCE	SPRINT POWER	TESTING	AEROBIC ENDURANCE	MUSCULAR FORCE	SPEED SKILLS	MUSCULAR ENDURANCE	ANAEROBIC ENDURANCE	SPRINT POWER	TESTING	AEROBIC ENDURANCE	MUSCULAR FORCE	SPEED SKILLS	MUSCULAR ENDURANCE	ANAEROBIC ENDURANCE	SPRINT POWER	TESTING
01	/																										
02	/																										
03	/																										
04	/																										
05	/																										
06	/																										
07	/																										
08	/																										
09	/																										
10	/																										
11	/																										
12	/																										
13	/																										
14	/																										
15	/																										
16	/																										
17	/																										
18	/																										
19	/																										
20	/																										
21	/																										
22	/																										
23	/																										
24	/																										
25	/																										
26	/																										

week	Mon.	races	pri.	period	vol.	WEIGHTS	swim							bike							run						
							AEROBIC ENDURANCE	MUSCULAR FORCE	SPEED SKILLS	MUSCULAR ENDURANCE	ANAEROBIC ENDURANCE	SPRINT POWER	TESTING	AEROBIC ENDURANCE	MUSCULAR FORCE	SPEED SKILLS	MUSCULAR ENDURANCE	ANAEROBIC ENDURANCE	SPRINT POWER	TESTING	AEROBIC ENDURANCE	MUSCULAR FORCE	SPEED SKILLS	MUSCULAR ENDURANCE	ANAEROBIC ENDURANCE	SPRINT POWER	TESTING
27	/																										
28	/																										
29	/																										
30	/																										
31	/																										
32	/																										
33	/																										
34	/																										
35	/																										
36	/																										
37	/																										
38	/																										
39	/																										
40	/																										
41	/																										
42	/																										
43	/																										
44	/																										
45	/																										
46	/																										
47	/																										
48	/																										
49	/																										
50	/																										
51	/																										
52	/																										

twelve-month calendar

period	month							weekly hours

period	month							weekly hours

period	month							weekly hours

period	month							weekly hours

period **month** **weekly hours**

weekly training hours

period	week	\begin{array}{c}\text{annual training hours}\end{array}									
		200	250	300	350	400	450	500	550	600	650
prep	all	3.5	4.0	5.0	6.0	7.0	7.5	8.5	9.0	10.0	11.0
base 1	1	4.0	5.0	6.0	7.0	8.0	9.0	10.0	11.0	12.0	12.5
	2	5.0	6.0	7.0	8.5	9.5	10.5	12.0	13.0	14.5	15.5
	3	5.5	6.5	8.0	9.5	10.5	12.0	13.5	14.5	16.0	17.5
	4	3.0	3.5	4.0	5.0	5.5	6.5	7.0	8.0	8.5	9.0
base 2	1	4.0	5.5	6.5	7.5	8.5	9.5	10.5	12.5	12.5	13.0
	2	5.0	6.5	7.5	9.0	10.0	11.5	12.5	14.0	15.0	16.5
	3	5.5	7.0	8.5	10.0	11.0	12.5	14.0	15.5	17.0	18.0
	4	3.0	3.5	4.5	5.0	5.5	6.5	7.0	8.0	8.5	9.0
base 3	1	4.5	5.5	7.0	8.0	9.0	10.0	11.0	12.5	13.5	14.5
	2	5.0	6.5	8.0	9.5	10.5	12.0	13.5	14.5	16.0	17.0
	3	6.0	7.5	9.0	10.5	11.5	13.0	15.0	16.5	18.0	19.0
	4	3.0	3.5	4.5	5.0	5.5	6.5	7.0	8.0	8.5	9.0
build 1	1	5.0	6.5	8.0	9.0	10.0	11.5	12.5	14.0	15.5	16.0
	2	5.0	6.5	8.0	9.0	10.0	11.5	12.5	14.0	15.5	16.0
	3	5.0	6.5	8.0	9.0	10.0	11.5	12.5	14.0	15.5	16.0
	4	3.0	3.5	4.5	5.0	5.5	6.5	7.0	8.0	8.5	9.0
build 2	1	5.0	6.0	7.0	8.5	9.5	10.5	12.0	13.0	14.5	15.5
	2	5.0	6.0	7.0	8.5	9.5	10.5	12.0	13.0	14.5	15.5
	3	5.0	6.0	7.0	8.5	9.5	10.5	12.0	13.0	14.5	15.5
	4	3.0	3.5	4.5	5.0	5.5	6.5	7.0	8.0	8.5	9.0
peak	1	4.0	5.5	6.5	7.5	8.5	9.5	10.5	11.5	13.0	13.5
	2	3.5	4.0	5.0	6.0	6.5	7.5	8.5	9.5	10.0	11.0
race	all	3.0	3.5	4.5	5.0	5.5	6.5	7.0	8.0	8.5	9.0
trans.	all	3.0	3.5	4.5	5.0	5.5	6.5	7.0	8.0	8.5	9.0

	annual training hours									
700	**750**	**800**	**850**	**900**	**950**	**1,000**	**1,050**	**1,100**	**1,150**	**1,200**
12.0	12.5	13.5	14.5	15.0	16.0	17.0	17.5	18.5	19.5	20.0
14.0	14.5	15.5	16.5	17.5	18.5	19.5	20.5	21.5	22.5	23.5
16.5	18.0	19.0	20.0	21.5	22.5	24.0	25.0	26.0	27.5	28.5
18.5	20.0	21.5	22.5	24.0	25.5	26.5	28.0	29.5	30.5	32.0
10.0	10.5	11.5	12.0	12.5	13.5	14.0	14.5	15.5	16.0	17.0
14.5	16.0	17.0	18.0	19.0	20.0	21.0	22.0	23.0	24.0	25.0
17.5	19.0	20.0	21.5	22.5	24.0	25.0	26.6	27.5	29.0	30.0
19.5	21.0	22.5	24.0	25.0	26.5	28.0	29.5	31.0	32.0	33.5
10.0	10.5	11.5	12.0	12.5	13.5	14.0	15.0	15.5	16.0	17.0
15.5	17.0	18.0	19.0	20.0	21.0	22.5	23.5	25.0	25.5	27.0
18.5	20.0	21.5	23.0	24.0	25.0	26.5	28.0	29.5	30.5	32.0
20.5	22.0	23.5	25.0	26.5	28.0	29.5	31.0	32.5	33.5	35.0
10.0	10.5	11.5	12.0	12.5	13.5	14.0	15.0	15.5	16.0	17.0
17.5	19.0	20.5	21.5	22.5	24.0	25.0	26.5	28.0	29.0	30.0
17.5	19.0	20.5	21.5	22.5	24.0	25.0	26.5	28.0	29.0	30.0
17.5	19.0	20.5	21.5	22.5	24.0	25.0	26.5	28.0	29.0	30.0
10.0	10.5	11.5	12.0	12.5	13.5	14.0	15.0	15.5	16.0	17.0
16.5	18.0	19.0	20.5	21.5	22.5	24.0	25.0	26.5	27.0	28.5
16.5	18.0	19.0	20.5	21.5	22.5	24.0	25.0	26.5	27.0	28.5
16.5	18.0	19.0	20.5	21.5	22.5	24.0	25.0	26.5	27.0	28.5
10.0	10.5	11.5	12.0	12.5	13.5	14.0	15.0	15.5	16.0	17.0
14.5	16.0	17.0	18.0	19.0	20.0	21.0	22.0	23.5	24.0	25.0
11.5	12.5	13.5	14.5	15.0	16.0	17.0	17.5	18.5	19.0	20.0
10.0	10.5	11.5	12.0	12.5	13.5	14.0	15.0	15.5	16.0	17.0
10.0	10.5	11.5	12.0	12.5	13.5	14.0	15.0	15.5	16.0	17.0

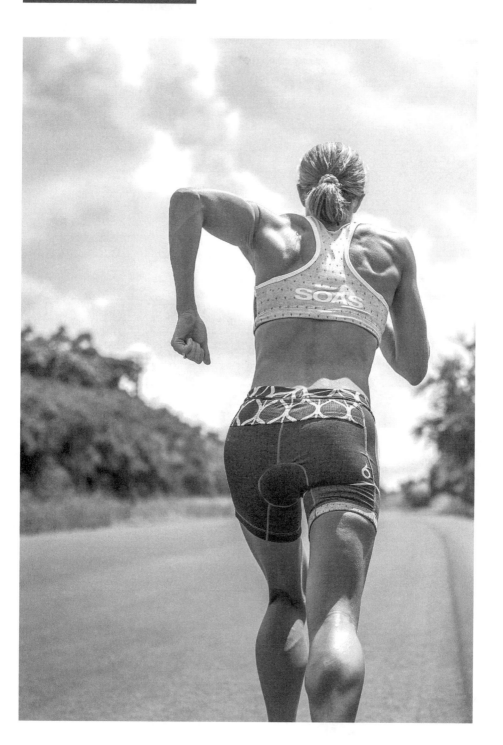

period: _____   planned hours: _____

MONDAY _____ / ____ / _____

▢ sleep ▢ fatigue ▢ stress ▢ soreness

resting heart rate_____ weight _____

WORKOUT 1 S B R O _____

planned workout _____

_____

route _____ dist. _____ time _____

avg. HR_____ avg. power _____

zone 1_____ 2_____ 3_____ 4_____ 5_____

WORKOUT 2 S B R O _____

planned workout _____

_____

route _____ dist. _____ time _____

avg. HR_____ avg. power _____

zone 1_____ 2_____ 3_____ 4_____ 5_____

notes _____

_____

_____

_____

_____

_____

_____

_____

_____

nutrition _____

_____

_____

_____

TUESDAY _____ / ____ / _____

▢ sleep ▢ fatigue ▢ stress ▢ soreness

resting heart rate_____ weight _____

WORKOUT 1 S B R O _____

planned workout _____

_____

route _____ dist. _____ time _____

avg. HR_____ avg. power _____

zone 1_____ 2_____ 3_____ 4_____ 5_____

WORKOUT 2 S B R O _____

planned workout _____

_____

route _____ dist. _____ time _____

avg. HR_____ avg. power _____

zone 1_____ 2_____ 3_____ 4_____ 5_____

notes _____

_____

_____

_____

_____

_____

_____

_____

_____

nutrition _____

_____

_____

_____

week goals: ▪ _____

▪ _____

▪ _____

WEDNESDAY ___ / ___ / ___

▪ sleep ▪ fatigue ▪ stress ▪ soreness

resting heart rate_____ weight _____

WORKOUT 1 S B R O _____

planned workout_____

_____

route _____dist. _____time _____

avg. HR_____avg. power_____

zone 1_____2_____3_____4_____5_____

WORKOUT 2 S B R O _____

planned workout_____

_____

route _____dist. _____time _____

avg. HR_____avg. power_____

zone 1_____2_____3_____4_____5_____

notes _____

_____

_____

_____

_____

_____

_____

_____

_____

_____

nutrition _____

_____

_____

_____

THURSDAY ___ / ___ / ___

▪ sleep ▪ fatigue ▪ stress ▪ soreness

resting heart rate_____ weight _____

WORKOUT 1 S B R O _____

planned workout_____

_____

route _____dist. _____time _____

avg. HR_____avg. power_____

zone 1_____2_____3_____4_____5_____

WORKOUT 2 S B R O _____

planned workout_____

_____

route _____dist. _____time _____

avg. HR_____avg. power_____

zone 1_____2_____3_____4_____5_____

notes _____

_____

_____

_____

_____

_____

_____

_____

_____

_____

nutrition _____

_____

_____

FRIDAY _____ / _____ / _____

☐ sleep ☐ fatigue ☐ stress ☐ soreness

resting heart rate_____ weight _____

WORKOUT 1 S B R O _____

planned workout _____

_____

_____

route _____ dist. _____ time _____

avg. HR _____ avg. power _____

zone 1_____ 2_____ 3_____ 4_____ 5_____

WORKOUT 2 S B R O _____

planned workout _____

_____

route _____ dist. _____ time _____

avg. HR _____ avg. power _____

zone 1_____ 2_____ 3_____ 4_____ 5_____

notes _____

_____
_____
_____
_____
_____
_____
_____
_____
_____

nutrition _____

_____
_____
_____

SATURDAY _____ / _____ / _____

☐ sleep ☐ fatigue ☐ stress ☐ soreness

resting heart rate_____ weight _____

WORKOUT 1 S B R O _____

planned workout _____

_____

_____

route _____ dist. _____ time _____

avg. HR _____ avg. power _____

zone 1_____ 2_____ 3_____ 4_____ 5_____

WORKOUT 2 S B R O _____

planned workout _____

_____

route _____ dist. _____ time _____

avg. HR _____ avg. power _____

zone 1_____ 2_____ 3_____ 4_____ 5_____

notes _____

_____
_____
_____
_____
_____
_____
_____
_____
_____

nutrition _____

_____
_____
_____

SUNDAY _____ / _____ / _____

■ sleep ■ fatigue ■ stress ■ soreness

resting heart rate_____ weight _____

WORKOUT 1 S B R O _____

planned workout_____

_____

_____

route _____ dist. _____ time _____

avg. HR_____ avg. power_____

zone 1_____ 2_____ 3_____ 4_____ 5_____

WORKOUT 2 S B R O _____

planned workout_____

_____

route _____ dist. _____ time _____

avg. HR_____ avg. power_____

zone 1_____ 2_____ 3_____ 4_____ 5_____

notes _____

_____

_____

_____

_____

_____

_____

_____

_____

_____

_____

nutrition _____

_____

_____

WEEKLY SUMMARY

	time	distance	YTD time	YTD distance
swim				
bike				
run				
strength				
other				
total				

notes

_____

_____

_____

_____

_____

_____

_____

_____

_____

period: _____   planned hours: _____

MONDAY _____ / _____ / _____   **notes** _____

☐ sleep ☐ fatigue ☐ stress ☐ soreness   _____

resting heart rate_____ weight _____   _____

WORKOUT 1 S B R O _____   _____

planned workout _____   _____

_____   _____

route _____ dist. _____ time _____   _____

avg. HR _____ avg. power _____   _____

zone 1____ 2____ 3____ 4____ 5____   _____

WORKOUT 2 S B R O _____   _____

planned workout _____   _____

_____   **nutrition** _____

route _____ dist. _____ time _____   _____

avg. HR _____ avg. power _____   _____

zone 1____ 2____ 3____ 4____ 5____   _____

TUESDAY _____ / _____ / _____   **notes** _____

☐ sleep ☐ fatigue ☐ stress ☐ soreness   _____

resting heart rate_____ weight _____   _____

WORKOUT 1 S B R O _____   _____

planned workout _____   _____

_____   _____

route _____ dist. _____ time _____   _____

avg. HR _____ avg. power _____   _____

zone 1____ 2____ 3____ 4____ 5____   _____

WORKOUT 2 S B R O _____   _____

planned workout _____   _____

_____   **nutrition** _____

route _____ dist. _____ time _____   _____

avg. HR _____ avg. power _____   _____

zone 1____ 2____ 3____ 4____ 5____   _____

week goals: ▪ _____

▪ _____

▪ _____

WEDNESDAY ____ / ____ / ____

▪ sleep ▪ fatigue ▪ stress ▪ soreness

resting heart rate_____ weight _____

WORKOUT 1 S B R O _____

planned workout_____

_____

route _____dist. _____time _____

avg. HR_____avg. power_____

zone 1_____ 2_____ 3_____ 4_____ 5_____

WORKOUT 2 S B R O _____

planned workout_____

_____

route _____dist. _____time _____

avg. HR_____avg. power_____

zone 1_____ 2_____ 3_____ 4_____ 5_____

notes _____

_____

_____

_____

_____

_____

_____

_____

_____

_____

_____

_____

nutrition _____

_____

_____

THURSDAY ____ / ____ / ____

▪ sleep ▪ fatigue ▪ stress ▪ soreness

resting heart rate_____ weight _____

WORKOUT 1 S B R O _____

planned workout_____

_____

route _____dist. _____time _____

avg. HR_____avg. power_____

zone 1_____ 2_____ 3_____ 4_____ 5_____

WORKOUT 2 S B R O _____

planned workout_____

_____

route _____dist. _____time _____

avg. HR_____avg. power_____

zone 1_____ 2_____ 3_____ 4_____ 5_____

notes _____

_____

_____

_____

_____

_____

_____

_____

_____

nutrition _____

_____

_____

FRIDAY _____ / _____ / _____

☐ sleep ☐ fatigue ☐ stress ☐ soreness

resting heart rate _____ weight _____

WORKOUT 1 S B R O _____

planned workout _____

_____

_____

route _____ dist. _____ time _____

avg. HR _____ avg. power _____

zone 1 _____ 2 _____ 3 _____ 4 _____ 5 _____

WORKOUT 2 S B R O _____

planned workout _____

_____

route _____ dist. _____ time _____

avg. HR _____ avg. power _____

zone 1 _____ 2 _____ 3 _____ 4 _____ 5 _____

notes _____

_____

_____

_____

_____

_____

_____

_____

_____

_____

_____

nutrition _____

_____

_____

_____

SATURDAY _____ / _____ / _____

☐ sleep ☐ fatigue ☐ stress ☐ soreness

resting heart rate _____ weight _____

WORKOUT 1 S B R O _____

planned workout _____

_____

_____

route _____ dist. _____ time _____

avg. HR _____ avg. power _____

zone 1 _____ 2 _____ 3 _____ 4 _____ 5 _____

WORKOUT 2 S B R O _____

planned workout _____

_____

_____

route _____ dist. _____ time _____

avg. HR _____ avg. power _____

zone 1 _____ 2 _____ 3 _____ 4 _____ 5 _____

notes _____

_____

_____

_____

_____

_____

_____

_____

_____

_____

nutrition _____

_____

_____

_____

SUNDAY _____ / ___ / _____

☐ sleep ☐ fatigue ☐ stress ☐ soreness

resting heart rate_____ weight _____

WORKOUT 1 S B R O _____

planned workout _____

_____

_____

route _____ dist. _____ time _____

avg. HR _____ avg. power _____

zone 1_____ 2_____ 3_____ 4_____ 5_____

WORKOUT 2 S B R O _____

planned workout _____

_____

route _____ dist. _____ time _____

avg. HR _____ avg. power _____

zone 1_____ 2_____ 3_____ 4_____ 5_____

notes _____

_____

_____

_____

_____

_____

_____

_____

_____

_____

_____

nutrition _____

_____

_____

_____

WEEKLY SUMMARY

	time	distance	YTD time	YTD distance
swim				
bike				
run				
strength				
other				
total				

notes

_____

_____

_____

_____

_____

_____

_____

_____

period: _____   planned hours: _____

MONDAY _____ / _____ /

■ sleep ■ fatigue ■ stress ■ soreness

resting heart rate_____ weight _____

WORKOUT 1 S B R O _____

planned workout _____

_____

route _____ dist. _____ time _____

avg. HR _____ avg. power _____

zone 1_____ 2_____ 3_____ 4_____ 5_____

WORKOUT 2 S B R O _____

planned workout _____

_____

route _____ dist. _____ time _____

avg. HR _____ avg. power _____

zone 1_____ 2_____ 3_____ 4_____ 5_____

notes _____

_____

_____

_____

_____

_____

_____

_____

_____

_____

_____

nutrition _____

_____

_____

_____

TUESDAY _____ / _____ /

■ sleep ■ fatigue ■ stress ■ soreness

resting heart rate_____ weight _____

WORKOUT 1 S B R O _____

planned workout _____

_____

route _____ dist. _____ time _____

avg. HR _____ avg. power _____

zone 1_____ 2_____ 3_____ 4_____ 5_____

WORKOUT 2 S B R O _____

planned workout _____

_____

route _____ dist. _____ time _____

avg. HR _____ avg. power _____

zone 1_____ 2_____ 3_____ 4_____ 5_____

notes _____

_____

_____

_____

_____

_____

_____

_____

_____

_____

_____

nutrition _____

_____

_____

week goals: ▪ _____

▪ _____

▪ _____

WEDNESDAY ____ / ____ / ____

▪ sleep ▪ fatigue ▪ stress ▪ soreness

resting heart rate_____ weight _____

WORKOUT 1 S B R O _____

planned workout _____

_____

route _____ dist. _____ time _____

avg. HR _____ avg. power _____

zone 1____ 2____ 3____ 4____ 5____

WORKOUT 2 S B R O _____

planned workout _____

_____

route _____ dist. _____ time _____

avg. HR _____ avg. power _____

zone 1____ 2____ 3____ 4____ 5____

notes _____

_____

_____

_____

_____

_____

_____

_____

_____

_____

_____

nutrition _____

_____

_____

_____

THURSDAY ____ / ____ / ____

▪ sleep ▪ fatigue ▪ stress ▪ soreness

resting heart rate_____ weight _____

WORKOUT 1 S B R O _____

planned workout _____

_____

route _____ dist. _____ time _____

avg. HR _____ avg. power _____

zone 1____ 2____ 3____ 4____ 5____

WORKOUT 2 S B R O _____

planned workout _____

_____

route _____ dist. _____ time _____

avg. HR _____ avg. power _____

zone 1____ 2____ 3____ 4____ 5____

notes _____

_____

_____

_____

_____

_____

_____

_____

_____

nutrition _____

_____

_____

_____

FRIDAY _____ / _____ /

□ sleep □ fatigue □ stress □ soreness

resting heart rate_____ weight _____

WORKOUT 1 S B R O _____

planned workout_____

_____

_____

route _____ dist. _____ time _____

avg. HR_____ avg. power _____

zone 1_____ 2_____ 3_____ 4_____ 5_____

WORKOUT 2 S B R O _____

planned workout_____

_____

route _____ dist. _____ time _____

avg. HR_____ avg. power _____

zone 1_____ 2_____ 3_____ 4_____ 5_____

notes _____

_____

_____

_____

_____

_____

_____

_____

_____

_____

nutrition _____

_____

_____

SATURDAY _____ / _____ /

□ sleep □ fatigue □ stress □ soreness

resting heart rate_____ weight _____

WORKOUT 1 S B R O _____

planned workout_____

_____

_____

route _____ dist. _____ time _____

avg. HR_____ avg. power _____

zone 1_____ 2_____ 3_____ 4_____ 5_____

WORKOUT 2 S B R O _____

planned workout_____

_____

_____

route _____ dist. _____ time _____

avg. HR_____ avg. power _____

zone 1_____ 2_____ 3_____ 4_____ 5_____

notes _____

_____

_____

_____

_____

_____

_____

_____

_____

_____

_____

nutrition _____

_____

_____

SUNDAY ____ / ____ / ____

☐ sleep ☐ fatigue ☐ stress ☐ soreness

resting heart rate _____ weight _____

WORKOUT 1 S B R O _____

planned workout _____

_____

_____

route _____ dist. _____ time _____

avg. HR _____ avg. power _____

zone 1 _____ 2 _____ 3 _____ 4 _____ 5 _____

WORKOUT 2 S B R O _____

planned workout _____

_____

route _____ dist. _____ time _____

avg. HR _____ avg. power _____

zone 1 _____ 2 _____ 3 _____ 4 _____ 5 _____

notes _____

_____

_____

_____

_____

_____

_____

_____

_____

nutrition _____

_____

_____

WEEKLY SUMMARY

	time	distance	YTD time	YTD distance
swim				
bike				
run				
strength				
other				
total				

notes

_____

_____

_____

_____

_____

_____

_____

_____

period: _____   planned hours: _____

MONDAY _____ / ____ / _____   **notes** _____

▢ sleep ▢ fatigue ▢ stress ▢ soreness   _____

resting heart rate _____ weight _____   _____

WORKOUT 1 S B R O _____   _____

planned workout _____   _____

_____   _____

route _____ dist. _____ time _____   _____

avg. HR _____ avg. power _____   _____

zone 1_____ 2_____ 3_____ 4_____ 5_____   _____

WORKOUT 2 S B R O _____   _____

planned workout _____   _____

_____   **nutrition** _____

route _____ dist. _____ time _____   _____

avg. HR _____ avg. power _____   _____

zone 1_____ 2_____ 3_____ 4_____ 5_____   _____

TUESDAY _____ / ____ / _____   **notes** _____

▢ sleep ▢ fatigue ▢ stress ▢ soreness   _____

resting heart rate _____ weight _____   _____

WORKOUT 1 S B R O _____   _____

planned workout _____   _____

_____   _____

route _____ dist. _____ time _____   _____

avg. HR _____ avg. power _____   _____

zone 1_____ 2_____ 3_____ 4_____ 5_____   _____

WORKOUT 2 S B R O _____   _____

planned workout _____   _____

_____   **nutrition** _____

route _____ dist. _____ time _____   _____

avg. HR _____ avg. power _____   _____

zone 1_____ 2_____ 3_____ 4_____ 5_____   _____

week goals: ▦ _____

▦ _____

▦ _____

WEDNESDAY _____ / _____ / _____

▦ sleep ▦ fatigue ▦ stress ▦ soreness

resting heart rate_____ weight _____

WORKOUT 1 S B R O _____

planned workout _____

_____

route _____ dist. _____ time _____

avg. HR _____ avg. power _____

zone 1_____ 2_____ 3_____ 4_____ 5_____

WORKOUT 2 S B R O _____

planned workout _____

_____

route _____ dist. _____ time _____

avg. HR _____ avg. power _____

zone 1_____ 2_____ 3_____ 4_____ 5_____

notes _____

_____

_____

_____

_____

_____

_____

_____

_____

_____

nutrition _____

_____

_____

THURSDAY _____ / _____ / _____

▦ sleep ▦ fatigue ▦ stress ▦ soreness

resting heart rate_____ weight _____

WORKOUT 1 S B R O _____

planned workout _____

_____

route _____ dist. _____ time _____

avg. HR _____ avg. power _____

zone 1_____ 2_____ 3_____ 4_____ 5_____

WORKOUT 2 S B R O _____

planned workout _____

_____

route _____ dist. _____ time _____

avg. HR _____ avg. power _____

zone 1_____ 2_____ 3_____ 4_____ 5_____

notes _____

_____

_____

_____

_____

_____

_____

_____

nutrition _____

_____

_____

FRIDAY _____ / /

■ sleep ■ fatigue ■ stress ■ soreness

resting heart rate_____ weight _____

WORKOUT 1 S B R O _____

planned workout_____

_____

_____

route _____dist. _____time _____

avg. HR_____avg. power_____

zone 1_____2_____3_____4_____5_____

WORKOUT 2 S B R O _____

planned workout_____

_____

route _____dist. _____time _____

avg. HR_____avg. power_____

zone 1_____2_____3_____4_____5_____

notes _____

_____

_____

_____

_____

_____

_____

_____

_____

nutrition _____

_____

_____

_____

SATURDAY _____ / /

■ sleep ■ fatigue ■ stress ■ soreness

resting heart rate_____ weight _____

WORKOUT 1 S B R O _____

planned workout_____

_____

_____

route _____dist. _____time _____

avg. HR_____avg. power_____

zone 1_____2_____3_____4_____5_____

WORKOUT 2 S B R O _____

planned workout_____

_____

route _____dist. _____time _____

avg. HR_____avg. power_____

zone 1_____2_____3_____4_____5_____

notes _____

_____

_____

_____

_____

_____

_____

_____

_____

nutrition _____

_____

_____

_____

SUNDAY _____ / _____ / _____

☐ sleep ☐ fatigue ☐ stress ☐ soreness

resting heart rate_____ weight _____

WORKOUT 1 S B R O _____

planned workout_____

_____

_____

route _____dist. _____time _____

avg. HR_____avg. power_____

zone 1_____2_____3_____4_____5_____

WORKOUT 2 S B R O _____

planned workout_____

_____

route _____dist. _____time _____

avg. HR_____avg. power_____

zone 1_____2_____3_____4_____5_____

notes _____

_____

_____

_____

_____

_____

_____

_____

_____

_____

nutrition _____

_____

_____

_____

WEEKLY SUMMARY

	time	distance	YTD time	YTD distance
swim				
bike				
run				
strength				
other				
total				

notes

_____

_____

_____

_____

_____

_____

_____

period: _____   planned hours: _____

MONDAY _____ / _____ / _____

☐ sleep ☐ fatigue ☐ stress ☐ soreness

resting heart rate_____ weight _____

WORKOUT 1 S B R O _____

planned workout _____

_____

route _____dist. _____time _____

avg. HR_____avg. power_____

zone 1_____2_____3_____4_____5_____

WORKOUT 2 S B R O _____

planned workout _____

_____

route _____dist. _____time _____

avg. HR_____avg. power_____

zone 1_____2_____3_____4_____5_____

notes _____

_____

_____

_____

_____

_____

_____

_____

_____

_____

nutrition _____

_____

_____

_____

TUESDAY _____ / _____ / _____

☐ sleep ☐ fatigue ☐ stress ☐ soreness

resting heart rate_____ weight _____

WORKOUT 1 S B R O _____

planned workout _____

_____

route _____dist. _____time _____

avg. HR_____avg. power_____

zone 1_____2_____3_____4_____5_____

WORKOUT 2 S B R O _____

planned workout _____

_____

route _____dist. _____time _____

avg. HR_____avg. power_____

zone 1_____2_____3_____4_____5_____

notes _____

_____

_____

_____

_____

_____

_____

_____

_____

nutrition _____

_____

_____

_____

week goals: ▪ _____

▪ _____

▪ _____

WEDNESDAY ____ / ____ / ____

▪ sleep ▪ fatigue ▪ stress ▪ soreness

resting heart rate_____ weight _____

WORKOUT 1 S B R O _____

planned workout_____

_____

route _____dist. _____time _____

avg. HR_____avg. power_____

zone 1_____2_____3_____4_____5_____

WORKOUT 2 S B R O _____

planned workout_____

_____

route _____dist. _____time _____

avg. HR_____avg. power_____

zone 1_____2_____3_____4_____5_____

notes _____

_____

_____

_____

_____

_____

_____

_____

_____

_____

nutrition _____

_____

_____

_____

THURSDAY ____ / ____ / ____

▪ sleep ▪ fatigue ▪ stress ▪ soreness

resting heart rate_____ weight _____

WORKOUT 1 S B R O _____

planned workout_____

_____

route _____dist. _____time _____

avg. HR_____avg. power_____

zone 1_____2_____3_____4_____5_____

WORKOUT 2 S B R O _____

planned workout_____

_____

route _____dist. _____time _____

avg. HR_____avg. power_____

zone 1_____2_____3_____4_____5_____

notes _____

_____

_____

_____

_____

_____

_____

_____

_____

_____

nutrition _____

_____

_____

_____

FRIDAY _____ / ___ /

■ sleep ■ fatigue ■ stress ■ soreness

resting heart rate_____ weight _____

WORKOUT 1 S B R O _____

planned workout_____

_____

_____

route _____ dist. _____ time _____

avg. HR_____ avg. power _____

zone 1_____ 2_____ 3_____ 4_____ 5_____

WORKOUT 2 S B R O _____

planned workout_____

_____

route _____ dist. _____ time _____

avg. HR_____ avg. power _____

zone 1_____ 2_____ 3_____ 4_____ 5_____

notes _____

_____

_____

_____

_____

_____

_____

_____

_____

_____

_____

nutrition _____

_____

_____

_____

SATURDAY _____ / ___ /

■ sleep ■ fatigue ■ stress ■ soreness

resting heart rate_____ weight _____

WORKOUT 1 S B R O _____

planned workout_____

_____

_____

route _____ dist. _____ time _____

avg. HR_____ avg. power _____

zone 1_____ 2_____ 3_____ 4_____ 5_____

WORKOUT 2 S B R O _____

planned workout_____

_____

route _____ dist. _____ time _____

avg. HR_____ avg. power _____

zone 1_____ 2_____ 3_____ 4_____ 5_____

notes _____

_____

_____

_____

_____

_____

_____

_____

_____

_____

_____

nutrition _____

_____

_____

SUNDAY _____ / _____ / _____

■ sleep ■ fatigue ■ stress ■ soreness

resting heart rate_____ weight _____

WORKOUT 1 S B R O _____

planned workout _____

_____

_____

route _____ dist. _____ time _____

avg. HR _____ avg. power _____

zone 1_____ 2_____ 3_____ 4_____ 5_____

WORKOUT 2 S B R O _____

planned workout _____

_____

route _____ dist. _____ time _____

avg. HR _____ avg. power _____

zone 1_____ 2_____ 3_____ 4_____ 5_____

notes _____

_____

_____

_____

_____

_____

_____

_____

_____

_____

nutrition _____

_____

_____

_____

WEEKLY SUMMARY

	time	distance	YTD time	YTD distance
swim				
bike				
run				
strength				
other				
total				

notes

_____

_____

_____

_____

_____

_____

_____

period: _____   planned hours: _____

MONDAY _____ / _____ / _____   **notes** _____

■ sleep ■ fatigue ■ stress ■ soreness   _____

resting heart rate_____ weight _____   _____

WORKOUT 1 S B R O _____   _____

planned workout _____   _____

_____   _____

route _____ dist. _____ time _____   _____

avg. HR _____ avg. power _____   _____

zone 1_____ 2_____ 3_____ 4_____ 5_____   _____

WORKOUT 2 S B R O _____   _____

planned workout _____   _____

_____   **nutrition** _____

route _____ dist. _____ time _____   _____

avg. HR _____ avg. power _____   _____

zone 1_____ 2_____ 3_____ 4_____ 5_____   _____

TUESDAY _____ / _____ / _____   **notes** _____

■ sleep ■ fatigue ■ stress ■ soreness   _____

resting heart rate_____ weight _____   _____

WORKOUT 1 S B R O _____   _____

planned workout _____   _____

_____   _____

route _____ dist. _____ time _____   _____

avg. HR _____ avg. power _____   _____

zone 1_____ 2_____ 3_____ 4_____ 5_____   _____

WORKOUT 2 S B R O _____   _____

planned workout _____   _____

_____   **nutrition** _____

route _____ dist. _____ time _____   _____

avg. HR _____ avg. power _____   _____

zone 1_____ 2_____ 3_____ 4_____ 5_____   _____

week goals: ▪ _____

▪ _____

▪ _____

WEDNESDAY ____ / ____ / ____

▪ sleep ▪ fatigue ▪ stress ▪ soreness

resting heart rate_____ weight _____

WORKOUT 1 S B R O _____

planned workout_____

_____

route _____dist. _____time _____

avg. HR_____avg. power_____

zone 1_____2_____3_____4_____5_____

WORKOUT 2 S B R O _____

planned workout_____

_____

route _____dist. _____time _____

avg. HR_____avg. power_____

zone 1_____2_____3_____4_____5_____

notes _____

_____

_____

_____

_____

_____

_____

_____

_____

_____

nutrition _____

_____

_____

_____

THURSDAY ____ / ____ / ____

▪ sleep ▪ fatigue ▪ stress ▪ soreness

resting heart rate_____ weight _____

WORKOUT 1 S B R O _____

planned workout_____

_____

route _____dist. _____time _____

avg. HR_____avg. power_____

zone 1_____2_____3_____4_____5_____

WORKOUT 2 S B R O _____

planned workout_____

_____

route _____dist. _____time _____

avg. HR_____avg. power_____

zone 1_____2_____3_____4_____5_____

notes _____

_____

_____

_____

_____

_____

_____

_____

_____

_____

nutrition _____

_____

_____

_____

FRIDAY ___ / ___ / ___

▢ sleep ▢ fatigue ▢ stress ▢ soreness

resting heart rate _____ weight _____

WORKOUT 1 S B R O _____

planned workout _____

_____

_____

route _____ dist. _____ time _____

avg. HR _____ avg. power _____

zone 1 ____ 2 ____ 3 ____ 4 ____ 5 ____

WORKOUT 2 S B R O _____

planned workout _____

_____

route _____ dist. _____ time _____

avg. HR _____ avg. power _____

zone 1 ____ 2 ____ 3 ____ 4 ____ 5 ____

notes _____

_____

_____

_____

_____

_____

_____

_____

_____

_____

_____

_____

nutrition _____

_____

_____

SATURDAY ___ / ___ / ___

▢ sleep ▢ fatigue ▢ stress ▢ soreness

resting heart rate _____ weight _____

WORKOUT 1 S B R O _____

planned workout _____

_____

_____

route _____ dist. _____ time _____

avg. HR _____ avg. power _____

zone 1 ____ 2 ____ 3 ____ 4 ____ 5 ____

WORKOUT 2 S B R O _____

planned workout _____

_____

_____

route _____ dist. _____ time _____

avg. HR _____ avg. power _____

zone 1 ____ 2 ____ 3 ____ 4 ____ 5 ____

notes _____

_____

_____

_____

_____

_____

_____

_____

_____

_____

_____

_____

nutrition _____

_____

_____

SUNDAY ___ / ___ / ___

☐ sleep ☐ fatigue ☐ stress ☐ soreness

resting heart rate _____ weight _____

WORKOUT 1 S B R O _____

planned workout _____

_____

_____

route _____ dist. _____ time _____

avg. HR _____ avg. power _____

zone 1____ 2____ 3____ 4____ 5____

WORKOUT 2 S B R O _____

planned workout _____

_____

route _____ dist. _____ time _____

avg. HR _____ avg. power _____

zone 1____ 2____ 3____ 4____ 5____

notes _____

_____

_____

_____

_____

_____

_____

_____

_____

_____

_____

_____

nutrition _____

_____

_____

_____

WEEKLY SUMMARY

	time	distance	YTD time	YTD distance
swim				
bike				
run				
strength				
other				
total				

notes

_____

_____

_____

_____

_____

_____

_____

_____

period: _____   planned hours: _____

MONDAY _____ / ____ / _____   **notes** _____

☐ sleep ☐ fatigue ☐ stress ☐ soreness   _____

resting heart rate _____ weight _____   _____

WORKOUT 1 S B R O _____   _____

planned workout _____   _____

_____   _____

route _____ dist. _____ time _____   _____

avg. HR _____ avg. power _____   _____

zone 1 ____ 2 ____ 3 ____ 4 ____ 5 ____   _____

WORKOUT 2 S B R O _____   _____

planned workout _____   _____

_____   **nutrition** _____

route _____ dist. _____ time _____   _____

avg. HR _____ avg. power _____   _____

zone 1 ____ 2 ____ 3 ____ 4 ____ 5 ____   _____

TUESDAY _____ / ____ / _____   **notes** _____

☐ sleep ☐ fatigue ☐ stress ☐ soreness   _____

resting heart rate _____ weight _____   _____

WORKOUT 1 S B R O _____   _____

planned workout _____   _____

_____   _____

route _____ dist. _____ time _____   _____

avg. HR _____ avg. power _____   _____

zone 1 ____ 2 ____ 3 ____ 4 ____ 5 ____   _____

WORKOUT 2 S B R O _____   _____

planned workout _____   _____

_____   **nutrition** _____

route _____ dist. _____ time _____   _____

avg. HR _____ avg. power _____   _____

zone 1 ____ 2 ____ 3 ____ 4 ____ 5 ____   _____

week goals: ▪ _____
▪ _____
▪ _____

WEDNESDAY ____/____/____

▪ sleep ▪ fatigue ▪ stress ▪ soreness

resting heart rate_____ weight _____

WORKOUT 1 S B R O _____

planned workout_____

_____

route _____dist. _____time _____

avg. HR_____avg. power_____

zone 1_____2_____ 3_____ 4_____ 5_____

WORKOUT 2 S B R O _____

planned workout_____

_____

route _____dist. _____time _____

avg. HR_____avg. power_____

zone 1_____2_____ 3_____ 4_____ 5_____

notes _____

_____
_____
_____
_____
_____
_____
_____
_____
_____

nutrition _____

_____
_____
_____

THURSDAY ____/____/____

▪ sleep ▪ fatigue ▪ stress ▪ soreness

resting heart rate_____ weight _____

WORKOUT 1 S B R O _____

planned workout_____

_____

route _____dist. _____time _____

avg. HR_____avg. power_____

zone 1_____2_____ 3_____ 4_____ 5_____

WORKOUT 2 S B R O _____

planned workout_____

_____

route _____dist. _____time _____

avg. HR_____avg. power_____

zone 1_____2_____ 3_____ 4_____ 5_____

notes _____

_____
_____
_____
_____
_____
_____
_____
_____
_____

nutrition _____

_____
_____
_____

FRIDAY ___ / ___ / ___

■ sleep ■ fatigue ■ stress ■ soreness

resting heart rate_____ weight _____

WORKOUT 1 S B R O _____

planned workout _____

_____

_____

route _____ dist. _____ time _____

avg. HR_____ avg. power _____

zone 1_____ 2_____ 3_____ 4_____ 5_____

WORKOUT 2 S B R O _____

planned workout _____

_____

route _____ dist. _____ time _____

avg. HR_____ avg. power _____

zone 1_____ 2_____ 3_____ 4_____ 5_____

notes _____

_____

_____

_____

_____

_____

_____

_____

_____

_____

nutrition _____

_____

_____

_____

SATURDAY ___ / ___ / ___

■ sleep ■ fatigue ■ stress ■ soreness

resting heart rate_____ weight _____

WORKOUT 1 S B R O _____

planned workout _____

_____

_____

route _____ dist. _____ time _____

avg. HR_____ avg. power _____

zone 1_____ 2_____ 3_____ 4_____ 5_____

WORKOUT 2 S B R O _____

planned workout _____

_____

_____

route _____ dist. _____ time _____

avg. HR_____ avg. power _____

zone 1_____ 2_____ 3_____ 4_____ 5_____

notes _____

_____

_____

_____

_____

_____

_____

_____

_____

_____

nutrition _____

_____

_____

_____

SUNDAY _____ / _____ / _____

- sleep - fatigue - stress - soreness

resting heart rate_____ weight _____

WORKOUT 1 S B R O _____

planned workout _____

_____

_____

route _____ dist. _____ time _____

avg. HR _____ avg. power _____

zone 1_____ 2_____ 3_____ 4_____ 5_____

WORKOUT 2 S B R O _____

planned workout _____

_____

route _____ dist. _____ time _____

avg. HR _____ avg. power _____

zone 1_____ 2_____ 3_____ 4_____ 5_____

notes _____

_____

_____

_____

_____

_____

_____

_____

_____

nutrition _____

_____

_____

_____

WEEKLY SUMMARY

	time	distance	YTD time	YTD distance
swim				
bike				
run				
strength				
other				
total				

notes

_____

_____

_____

_____

_____

_____

_____

_____

period: _____   planned hours: _____

MONDAY _____ / _____ / _____   **notes** _____

■ sleep ■ fatigue ■ stress ■ soreness   _____

resting heart rate_____ weight _____   _____

WORKOUT 1 S B R O _____   _____

planned workout _____   _____

_____   _____

route _____ dist. _____ time _____   _____

avg. HR _____ avg. power _____   _____

zone 1_____ 2_____ 3_____ 4_____ 5_____   _____

WORKOUT 2 S B R O _____   _____

planned workout _____   _____

_____   **nutrition** _____

route _____ dist. _____ time _____   _____

avg. HR _____ avg. power _____   _____

zone 1_____ 2_____ 3_____ 4_____ 5_____   _____

TUESDAY _____ / _____ / _____   **notes** _____

■ sleep ■ fatigue ■ stress ■ soreness   _____

resting heart rate_____ weight _____   _____

WORKOUT 1 S B R O _____   _____

planned workout _____   _____

_____   _____

route _____ dist. _____ time _____   _____

avg. HR _____ avg. power _____   _____

zone 1_____ 2_____ 3_____ 4_____ 5_____   _____

WORKOUT 2 S B R O _____   _____

planned workout _____   _____

_____   **nutrition** _____

route _____ dist. _____ time _____   _____

avg. HR _____ avg. power _____   _____

zone 1_____ 2_____ 3_____ 4_____ 5_____   _____

week goals: ■ _____

■ _____

■ _____

WEDNESDAY ____ / ____ / ____

■ sleep ■ fatigue ■ stress ■ soreness

resting heart rate_____ weight _____

WORKOUT 1 S B R O _____

planned workout_____

_____

route _____ dist. _____ time _____

avg. HR_____ avg. power _____

zone 1_____ 2_____ 3_____ 4_____ 5_____

WORKOUT 2 S B R O _____

planned workout_____

_____

route _____ dist. _____ time _____

avg. HR_____ avg. power _____

zone 1_____ 2_____ 3_____ 4_____ 5_____

notes _____

_____

_____

_____

_____

_____

_____

_____

_____

_____

nutrition _____

_____

_____

_____

THURSDAY ____ / ____ / ____

■ sleep ■ fatigue ■ stress ■ soreness

resting heart rate_____ weight _____

WORKOUT 1 S B R O _____

planned workout_____

_____

route _____ dist. _____ time _____

avg. HR_____ avg. power _____

zone 1_____ 2_____ 3_____ 4_____ 5_____

WORKOUT 2 S B R O _____

planned workout_____

_____

route _____ dist. _____ time _____

avg. HR_____ avg. power _____

zone 1_____ 2_____ 3_____ 4_____ 5_____

notes _____

_____

_____

_____

_____

_____

_____

_____

_____

_____

nutrition _____

_____

_____

_____

FRIDAY ___ / ___ / ___

☐ sleep ☐ fatigue ☐ stress ☐ soreness

resting heart rate _____ weight _____

WORKOUT 1 S B R O _____

planned workout _____

_____

_____

route _____ dist. _____ time _____

avg. HR _____ avg. power _____

zone 1 ____ 2 ____ 3 ____ 4 ____ 5 ____

WORKOUT 2 S B R O _____

planned workout _____

_____

route _____ dist. _____ time _____

avg. HR _____ avg. power _____

zone 1 ____ 2 ____ 3 ____ 4 ____ 5 ____

notes _____

_____

_____

_____

_____

_____

_____

_____

_____

_____

_____

nutrition _____

_____

_____

SATURDAY ___ / ___ / ___

☐ sleep ☐ fatigue ☐ stress ☐ soreness

resting heart rate _____ weight _____

WORKOUT 1 S B R O _____

planned workout _____

_____

_____

route _____ dist. _____ time _____

avg. HR _____ avg. power _____

zone 1 ____ 2 ____ 3 ____ 4 ____ 5 ____

WORKOUT 2 S B R O _____

planned workout _____

_____

route _____ dist. _____ time _____

avg. HR _____ avg. power _____

zone 1 ____ 2 ____ 3 ____ 4 ____ 5 ____

notes _____

_____

_____

_____

_____

_____

_____

_____

_____

_____

nutrition _____

_____

_____

SUNDAY ___/___/___

☐ sleep ☐ fatigue ☐ stress ☐ soreness

resting heart rate_____ weight _____

WORKOUT 1 S B R O _____

planned workout_____

_____

_____

route _____ dist. _____ time _____

avg. HR_____ avg. power _____

zone 1_____ 2_____ 3_____ 4_____ 5_____

WORKOUT 2 S B R O _____

planned workout_____

_____

route _____ dist. _____ time _____

avg. HR_____ avg. power _____

zone 1_____ 2_____ 3_____ 4_____ 5_____

notes _____

_____

_____

_____

_____

_____

_____

_____

_____

_____

_____

nutrition _____

_____

_____

_____

WEEKLY SUMMARY

	time	distance	YTD time	YTD distance
swim				
bike				
run				
strength				
other				
total				

notes

_____

_____

_____

_____

_____

_____

_____

_____

period: _____   planned hours: _____

MONDAY _____ / ____ / _____   **notes** _____

■ sleep ■ fatigue ■ stress ■ soreness   _____

resting heart rate_____ weight _____   _____

WORKOUT 1 S B R O _____   _____

planned workout _____   _____

_____   _____

route _____ dist. _____ time _____   _____

avg. HR _____ avg. power _____   _____

zone 1____ 2____ 3____ 4____ 5____   _____

WORKOUT 2 S B R O _____   _____

planned workout _____   _____

_____   **nutrition** _____

route _____ dist. _____ time _____   _____

avg. HR _____ avg. power _____   _____

zone 1____ 2____ 3____ 4____ 5____   _____

TUESDAY _____ / ____ / _____   **notes** _____

■ sleep ■ fatigue ■ stress ■ soreness   _____

resting heart rate_____ weight _____   _____

WORKOUT 1 S B R O _____   _____

planned workout _____   _____

_____   _____

route _____ dist. _____ time _____   _____

avg. HR _____ avg. power _____   _____

zone 1____ 2____ 3____ 4____ 5____   _____

WORKOUT 2 S B R O _____   _____

planned workout _____   _____

_____   **nutrition** _____

route _____ dist. _____ time _____   _____

avg. HR _____ avg. power _____   _____

zone 1____ 2____ 3____ 4____ 5____   _____

week goals: ▪ _____

▪ _____

▪ _____

WEDNESDAY ____/____/____

▪ sleep ▪ fatigue ▪ stress ▪ soreness

resting heart rate_____weight _____

WORKOUT 1 S B R O _____

planned workout_____

_____

route _____dist. _____time _____

avg. HR_____avg. power_____

zone 1_____2_____3_____4_____5_____

WORKOUT 2 S B R O _____

planned workout_____

_____

route _____dist. _____time _____

avg. HR_____avg. power_____

zone 1_____2_____3_____4_____5_____

notes _____

_____

_____

_____

_____

_____

_____

_____

_____

_____

nutrition _____

_____

_____

_____

THURSDAY ____/____/____

▪ sleep ▪ fatigue ▪ stress ▪ soreness

resting heart rate_____weight _____

WORKOUT 1 S B R O _____

planned workout_____

_____

route _____dist. _____time _____

avg. HR_____avg. power_____

zone 1_____2_____3_____4_____5_____

WORKOUT 2 S B R O _____

planned workout_____

_____

route _____dist. _____time _____

avg. HR_____avg. power_____

zone 1_____2_____3_____4_____5_____

notes _____

_____

_____

_____

_____

_____

_____

_____

_____

nutrition _____

_____

_____

_____

FRIDAY _____ / _____ / _____

☐ sleep ☐ fatigue ☐ stress ☐ soreness

resting heart rate _____ weight _____

WORKOUT 1 S B R O _____

planned workout _____
_____
_____

route _____ dist. _____ time _____

avg. HR _____ avg. power _____

zone 1 ____ 2 ____ 3 ____ 4 ____ 5 ____

WORKOUT 2 S B R O _____

planned workout _____
_____

route _____ dist. _____ time _____

avg. HR _____ avg. power _____

zone 1 ____ 2 ____ 3 ____ 4 ____ 5 ____

notes _____
_____
_____
_____
_____
_____
_____
_____
_____
_____
_____
_____

nutrition _____
_____
_____
_____

SATURDAY _____ / _____ / _____

☐ sleep ☐ fatigue ☐ stress ☐ soreness

resting heart rate _____ weight _____

WORKOUT 1 S B R O _____

planned workout _____
_____
_____

route _____ dist. _____ time _____

avg. HR _____ avg. power _____

zone 1 ____ 2 ____ 3 ____ 4 ____ 5 ____

WORKOUT 2 S B R O _____

planned workout _____
_____
_____

route _____ dist. _____ time _____

avg. HR _____ avg. power _____

zone 1 ____ 2 ____ 3 ____ 4 ____ 5 ____

notes _____
_____
_____
_____
_____
_____
_____
_____
_____
_____
_____

nutrition _____
_____
_____

SUNDAY _____ / ___ / _____

◻ sleep ◻ fatigue ◻ stress ◻ soreness

resting heart rate_____ weight _____

WORKOUT 1 S B R O _____

planned workout _____

_____

_____

route _____dist. _____time _____

avg. HR_____avg. power_____

zone 1_____2_____3_____4_____5_____

WORKOUT 2 S B R O _____

planned workout _____

_____

route _____dist. _____time _____

avg. HR_____avg. power_____

zone 1_____2_____3_____4_____5_____

notes _____

_____

_____

_____

_____

_____

_____

_____

_____

_____

_____

_____

nutrition _____

_____

_____

_____

WEEKLY SUMMARY

	time	distance	YTD time	YTD distance
swim				
bike				
run				
strength				
other				
total				

notes

_____

_____

_____

_____

_____

_____

_____

_____

period: _____   planned hours: _____

MONDAY _____ / _____ / _____

▨ sleep ▨ fatigue ▨ stress ▨ soreness

resting heart rate_____ weight _____

WORKOUT 1 S B R 0 _____

planned workout _____

_____

route _____ dist. _____ time _____

avg. HR _____ avg. power _____

zone 1_____ 2_____ 3_____ 4_____ 5_____

WORKOUT 2 S B R 0 _____

planned workout _____

_____

route _____ dist. _____ time _____

avg. HR _____ avg. power _____

zone 1_____ 2_____ 3_____ 4_____ 5_____

notes _____

_____

_____

_____

_____

_____

_____

_____

_____

nutrition _____

_____

_____

_____

TUESDAY _____ / _____ / _____

▨ sleep ▨ fatigue ▨ stress ▨ soreness

resting heart rate_____ weight _____

WORKOUT 1 S B R 0 _____

planned workout _____

_____

route _____ dist. _____ time _____

avg. HR _____ avg. power _____

zone 1_____ 2_____ 3_____ 4_____ 5_____

WORKOUT 2 S B R 0 _____

planned workout _____

_____

route _____ dist. _____ time _____

avg. HR _____ avg. power _____

zone 1_____ 2_____ 3_____ 4_____ 5_____

notes _____

_____

_____

_____

_____

_____

_____

_____

_____

nutrition _____

_____

_____

_____

week goals: ■ _____
■ _____
■ _____

WEDNESDAY ___ / ___ / ___

■ sleep   ■ fatigue   ■ stress   ■ soreness

resting heart rate_____ weight _____

WORKOUT 1   S B R O _____

planned workout_____

_____

route _____ dist. _____ time _____

avg. HR_____ avg. power _____

zone 1_____ 2_____ 3_____ 4_____ 5_____

WORKOUT 2   S B R O _____

planned workout_____

_____

route _____ dist. _____ time _____

avg. HR_____ avg. power _____

zone 1_____ 2_____ 3_____ 4_____ 5_____

notes _____
_____
_____
_____
_____
_____
_____
_____
_____

nutrition _____
_____
_____
_____

THURSDAY ___ / ___ / ___

■ sleep   ■ fatigue   ■ stress   ■ soreness

resting heart rate_____ weight _____

WORKOUT 1   S B R O _____

planned workout_____

_____

route _____ dist. _____ time _____

avg. HR_____ avg. power _____

zone 1_____ 2_____ 3_____ 4_____ 5_____

WORKOUT 2   S B R O _____

planned workout_____

_____

route _____ dist. _____ time _____

avg. HR_____ avg. power _____

zone 1_____ 2_____ 3_____ 4_____ 5_____

notes _____
_____
_____
_____
_____
_____
_____
_____
_____

nutrition _____
_____
_____
_____

FRIDAY ___ / ___ / ___

☐ sleep ☐ fatigue ☐ stress ☐ soreness

resting heart rate _____ weight _____

WORKOUT 1 S B R O _____

planned workout _____

_____

_____

route _____ dist. _____ time _____

avg. HR _____ avg. power _____

zone 1 ___ 2 ___ 3 ___ 4 ___ 5 ___

WORKOUT 2 S B R O _____

planned workout _____

_____

route _____ dist. _____ time _____

avg. HR _____ avg. power _____

zone 1 ___ 2 ___ 3 ___ 4 ___ 5 ___

notes _____

_____

_____

_____

_____

_____

_____

_____

_____

_____

nutrition _____

_____

_____

_____

SATURDAY ___ / ___ / ___

☐ sleep ☐ fatigue ☐ stress ☐ soreness

resting heart rate _____ weight _____

WORKOUT 1 S B R O _____

planned workout _____

_____

_____

route _____ dist. _____ time _____

avg. HR _____ avg. power _____

zone 1 ___ 2 ___ 3 ___ 4 ___ 5 ___

WORKOUT 2 S B R O _____

planned workout _____

_____

_____

route _____ dist. _____ time _____

avg. HR _____ avg. power _____

zone 1 ___ 2 ___ 3 ___ 4 ___ 5 ___

notes _____

_____

_____

_____

_____

_____

_____

_____

_____

_____

_____

nutrition _____

_____

_____

SUNDAY _____ / _____ / _____

▢ sleep ▢ fatigue ▢ stress ▢ soreness

resting heart rate _____ weight _____

WORKOUT 1 S B R O _____

planned workout _____

_____

_____

route _____ dist. _____ time _____

avg. HR _____ avg. power _____

zone 1 _____ 2 _____ 3 _____ 4 _____ 5 _____

WORKOUT 2 S B R O _____

planned workout _____

_____

route _____ dist. _____ time _____

avg. HR _____ avg. power _____

zone 1 _____ 2 _____ 3 _____ 4 _____ 5 _____

notes _____

_____

_____

_____

_____

_____

_____

_____

_____

_____

nutrition _____

_____

_____

_____

WEEKLY SUMMARY

	time	distance	YTD time	YTD distance
swim				
bike				
run				
strength				
other				
total				

notes

_____

_____

_____

_____

_____

_____

_____

_____

period: _____   planned hours: _____

MONDAY _____ / ____ / _____

▨ sleep ▨ fatigue ▨ stress ▨ soreness

resting heart rate_____ weight _____

WORKOUT 1 S B R O _____

planned workout_____

_____

route _____ dist. _____ time _____

avg. HR_____ avg. power_____

zone 1____ 2____ 3____ 4____ 5____

WORKOUT 2 S B R O _____

planned workout_____

_____

route _____ dist. _____ time _____

avg. HR_____ avg. power_____

zone 1____ 2____ 3____ 4____ 5____

notes _____

_____

_____

_____

_____

_____

_____

_____

_____

_____

_____

nutrition _____

_____

_____

_____

TUESDAY _____ / ____ / _____

▨ sleep ▨ fatigue ▨ stress ▨ soreness

resting heart rate_____ weight _____

WORKOUT 1 S B R O _____

planned workout_____

_____

route _____ dist. _____ time _____

avg. HR_____ avg. power_____

zone 1____ 2____ 3____ 4____ 5____

WORKOUT 2 S B R O _____

planned workout_____

_____

route _____ dist. _____ time _____

avg. HR_____ avg. power_____

zone 1____ 2____ 3____ 4____ 5____

notes _____

_____

_____

_____

_____

_____

_____

_____

_____

nutrition _____

_____

_____

_____

week goals: ■ _____
■ _____
■ _____

WEDNESDAY _____ / _____ / _____

■ sleep ■ fatigue ■ stress ■ soreness

resting heart rate_____ weight _____

WORKOUT 1 S B R O _____

planned workout _____

_____

route _____ dist. _____ time _____

avg. HR _____ avg. power _____

zone 1_____ 2_____ 3_____ 4_____ 5_____

WORKOUT 2 S B R O _____

planned workout _____

_____

route _____ dist. _____ time _____

avg. HR _____ avg. power _____

zone 1_____ 2_____ 3_____ 4_____ 5_____

notes _____
_____
_____
_____
_____
_____
_____
_____
_____
_____
_____

nutrition _____
_____
_____
_____

THURSDAY _____ / _____ / _____

■ sleep ■ fatigue ■ stress ■ soreness

resting heart rate_____ weight _____

WORKOUT 1 S B R O _____

planned workout _____

_____

route _____ dist. _____ time _____

avg. HR _____ avg. power _____

zone 1_____ 2_____ 3_____ 4_____ 5_____

WORKOUT 2 S B R O _____

planned workout _____

_____

route _____ dist. _____ time _____

avg. HR _____ avg. power _____

zone 1_____ 2_____ 3_____ 4_____ 5_____

notes _____
_____
_____
_____
_____
_____
_____
_____
_____
_____
_____

nutrition _____
_____
_____
_____

FRIDAY ___/___/___

▢ sleep ▢ fatigue ▢ stress ▢ soreness

resting heart rate_____ weight_____

WORKOUT 1 S B R O _____

planned workout _____

_____

_____

route _____ dist. _____ time _____

avg. HR _____ avg. power _____

zone 1____ 2____ 3____ 4____ 5____

WORKOUT 2 S B R O _____

planned workout _____

_____

route _____ dist. _____ time _____

avg. HR _____ avg. power _____

zone 1____ 2____ 3____ 4____ 5____

notes _____

_____

_____

_____

_____

_____

_____

_____

_____

_____

_____

nutrition _____

_____

_____

_____

SATURDAY ___/___/___

▢ sleep ▢ fatigue ▢ stress ▢ soreness

resting heart rate_____ weight_____

WORKOUT 1 S B R O _____

planned workout _____

_____

_____

route _____ dist. _____ time _____

avg. HR _____ avg. power _____

zone 1____ 2____ 3____ 4____ 5____

WORKOUT 2 S B R O _____

planned workout _____

_____

_____

route _____ dist. _____ time _____

avg. HR _____ avg. power _____

zone 1____ 2____ 3____ 4____ 5____

notes _____

_____

_____

_____

_____

_____

_____

_____

_____

nutrition _____

_____

_____

SUNDAY ____ / ___ / _____

☐ sleep ☐ fatigue ☐ stress ☐ soreness

resting heart rate_____ weight _____

WORKOUT 1 S B R O _____

planned workout_____

_____

_____

route _____dist. _____time _____

avg. HR_____avg. power_____

zone 1_____ 2_____ 3_____ 4_____ 5_____

WORKOUT 2 S B R O _____

planned workout_____

_____

route _____dist. _____time _____

avg. HR_____avg. power_____

zone 1_____ 2_____ 3_____ 4_____ 5_____

notes _____

_____

_____

_____

_____

_____

_____

_____

_____

_____

_____

nutrition _____

_____

_____

_____

WEEKLY SUMMARY

	time	distance	YTD time	YTD distance
swim				
bike				
run				
strength				
other				
total				

notes

_____

_____

_____

_____

_____

_____

_____

_____

_____

period: _____   planned hours: _____

MONDAY _____ / ____ / _____   **notes** _____

☐ sleep ☐ fatigue ☐ stress ☐ soreness   _____

resting heart rate_____ weight _____   _____

WORKOUT 1 S B R O _____   _____

planned workout_____   _____

_____   _____

route _____dist. _____time _____   _____

avg. HR_____avg. power_____   _____

zone 1_____2_____3_____4_____5_____   _____

WORKOUT 2 S B R O _____   _____

planned workout_____   _____

_____   **nutrition** _____

route _____dist. _____time _____   _____

avg. HR_____avg. power_____   _____

zone 1_____2_____3_____4_____5_____   _____

TUESDAY _____ / ____ / _____   **notes** _____

☐ sleep ☐ fatigue ☐ stress ☐ soreness   _____

resting heart rate_____ weight _____   _____

WORKOUT 1 S B R O _____   _____

planned workout_____   _____

_____   _____

route _____dist. _____time _____   _____

avg. HR_____avg. power_____   _____

zone 1_____2_____3_____4_____5_____   _____

WORKOUT 2 S B R O _____   _____

planned workout_____   _____

_____   **nutrition** _____

route _____dist. _____time _____   _____

avg. HR_____avg. power_____   _____

zone 1_____2_____3_____4_____5_____   _____

week goals: ▪ _____

▪ _____

▪ _____

WEDNESDAY _____ / _____ / _____

▪ sleep ▪ fatigue ▪ stress ▪ soreness

resting heart rate _____ weight _____

WORKOUT 1 S B R O _____

planned workout _____

_____

route _____ dist. _____ time _____

avg. HR _____ avg. power _____

zone 1 _____ 2 _____ 3 _____ 4 _____ 5 _____

WORKOUT 2 S B R O _____

planned workout _____

_____

route _____ dist. _____ time _____

avg. HR _____ avg. power _____

zone 1 _____ 2 _____ 3 _____ 4 _____ 5 _____

notes _____

_____

_____

_____

_____

_____

_____

_____

_____

nutrition _____

_____

_____

_____

THURSDAY _____ / _____ / _____

▪ sleep ▪ fatigue ▪ stress ▪ soreness

resting heart rate _____ weight _____

WORKOUT 1 S B R O _____

planned workout _____

_____

route _____ dist. _____ time _____

avg. HR _____ avg. power _____

zone 1 _____ 2 _____ 3 _____ 4 _____ 5 _____

WORKOUT 2 S B R O _____

planned workout _____

_____

route _____ dist. _____ time _____

avg. HR _____ avg. power _____

zone 1 _____ 2 _____ 3 _____ 4 _____ 5 _____

notes _____

_____

_____

_____

_____

_____

_____

_____

_____

nutrition _____

_____

_____

_____

FRIDAY ___ / ___ / ___

□ sleep □ fatigue □ stress □ soreness

resting heart rate ___ weight ___

WORKOUT 1 S B R O ___

planned workout ___

___

___

route ___ dist. ___ time ___

avg. HR ___ avg. power ___

zone 1 ___ 2 ___ 3 ___ 4 ___ 5 ___

WORKOUT 2 S B R O ___

planned workout ___

___

route ___ dist. ___ time ___

avg. HR ___ avg. power ___

zone 1 ___ 2 ___ 3 ___ 4 ___ 5 ___

notes ___

___
___
___
___
___
___
___
___
___

nutrition ___

___
___
___

SATURDAY ___ / ___ / ___

□ sleep □ fatigue □ stress □ soreness

resting heart rate ___ weight ___

WORKOUT 1 S B R O ___

planned workout ___

___

___

route ___ dist. ___ time ___

avg. HR ___ avg. power ___

zone 1 ___ 2 ___ 3 ___ 4 ___ 5 ___

WORKOUT 2 S B R O ___

planned workout ___

___

route ___ dist. ___ time ___

avg. HR ___ avg. power ___

zone 1 ___ 2 ___ 3 ___ 4 ___ 5 ___

notes ___

___
___
___
___
___
___
___
___

nutrition ___

___
___

SUNDAY _____ / ____ / _____

☐ sleep ☐ fatigue ☐ stress ☐ soreness

resting heart rate_____weight_____

WORKOUT 1 S B R O _____

planned workout _____

_____

_____

route _____ dist. _____ time _____

avg. HR _____ avg. power _____

zone 1_____ 2_____ 3_____ 4_____ 5_____

WORKOUT 2 S B R O _____

planned workout _____

_____

route _____ dist. _____ time _____

avg. HR _____ avg. power _____

zone 1_____ 2_____ 3_____ 4_____ 5_____

notes _____

_____

_____

_____

_____

_____

_____

_____

_____

_____

_____

_____

nutrition _____

_____

_____

WEEKLY SUMMARY

	time	distance	YTD time	YTD distance
swim				
bike				
run				
strength				
other				
total				

notes

_____

_____

_____

_____

_____

_____

_____

_____

_____

period: _____ planned hours: _____

MONDAY ____ / ____ / ____

☐ sleep ☐ fatigue ☐ stress ☐ soreness

resting heart rate_____ weight _____

WORKOUT 1 S B R O _____

planned workout _____

_____

route _____ dist. _____ time _____

avg. HR _____ avg. power _____

zone 1____ 2____ 3____ 4____ 5____

WORKOUT 2 S B R O _____

planned workout _____

_____

route _____ dist. _____ time _____

avg. HR _____ avg. power _____

zone 1____ 2____ 3____ 4____ 5____

notes _____
_____
_____
_____
_____
_____
_____
_____
_____
_____

nutrition _____
_____
_____
_____

TUESDAY ____ / ____ / ____

☐ sleep ☐ fatigue ☐ stress ☐ soreness

resting heart rate_____ weight _____

WORKOUT 1 S B R O _____

planned workout _____

_____

route _____ dist. _____ time _____

avg. HR _____ avg. power _____

zone 1____ 2____ 3____ 4____ 5____

WORKOUT 2 S B R O _____

planned workout _____

_____

route _____ dist. _____ time _____

avg. HR _____ avg. power _____

zone 1____ 2____ 3____ 4____ 5____

notes _____
_____
_____
_____
_____
_____
_____
_____
_____
_____

nutrition _____
_____
_____
_____

week goals: ▣ _____

▣ _____

▣ _____

WEDNESDAY ____ / ____ / ____

▣ sleep ▣ fatigue ▣ stress ▣ soreness

resting heart rate_____ weight _____

WORKOUT 1 S B R O _____

planned workout _____

_____

route _____ dist. _____ time _____

avg. HR _____ avg. power _____

zone 1____ 2____ 3____ 4____ 5____

WORKOUT 2 S B R O _____

planned workout _____

_____

route _____ dist. _____ time _____

avg. HR _____ avg. power _____

zone 1____ 2____ 3____ 4____ 5____

notes _____

_____

_____

_____

_____

_____

_____

_____

_____

_____

_____

nutrition _____

_____

_____

_____

THURSDAY ____ / ____ / ____

▣ sleep ▣ fatigue ▣ stress ▣ soreness

resting heart rate_____ weight _____

WORKOUT 1 S B R O _____

planned workout _____

_____

route _____ dist. _____ time _____

avg. HR _____ avg. power _____

zone 1____ 2____ 3____ 4____ 5____

WORKOUT 2 S B R O _____

planned workout _____

_____

route _____ dist. _____ time _____

avg. HR _____ avg. power _____

zone 1____ 2____ 3____ 4____ 5____

notes _____

_____

_____

_____

_____

_____

_____

_____

_____

_____

_____

nutrition _____

_____

_____

_____

FRIDAY _____ / ___ /

sleep fatigue stress soreness

resting heart rate_____ weight _____

WORKOUT 1 S B R O _____

planned workout _____

_____

_____

route _____ dist. _____ time _____

avg. HR _____ avg. power _____

zone 1_____ 2_____ 3_____ 4_____ 5_____

WORKOUT 2 S B R O _____

planned workout _____

_____

route _____ dist. _____ time _____

avg. HR _____ avg. power _____

zone 1_____ 2_____ 3_____ 4_____ 5_____

notes _____

_____

_____

_____

_____

_____

_____

_____

_____

_____

_____

_____

nutrition _____

_____

_____

_____

SATURDAY _____ / ___ /

sleep fatigue stress soreness

resting heart rate_____ weight _____

WORKOUT 1 S B R O _____

planned workout _____

_____

_____

route _____ dist. _____ time _____

avg. HR _____ avg. power _____

zone 1_____ 2_____ 3_____ 4_____ 5_____

WORKOUT 2 S B R O _____

planned workout _____

_____

route _____ dist. _____ time _____

avg. HR _____ avg. power _____

zone 1_____ 2_____ 3_____ 4_____ 5_____

notes _____

_____

_____

_____

_____

_____

_____

_____

_____

_____

_____

nutrition _____

_____

_____

_____

SUNDAY _____ / ___ / ___

sleep ▨ fatigue ▨ stress ▨ soreness

resting heart rate_____ weight _____

WORKOUT 1 S B R O _____

planned workout_____

_____

_____

route _____ dist. _____ time _____

avg. HR_____ avg. power _____

zone 1_____ 2_____ 3_____ 4_____ 5_____

WORKOUT 2 S B R O _____

planned workout_____

_____

route _____ dist. _____ time _____

avg. HR_____ avg. power _____

zone 1_____ 2_____ 3_____ 4_____ 5_____

notes _____

_____

_____

_____

_____

_____

_____

_____

_____

_____

_____

_____

nutrition _____

_____

_____

_____

WEEKLY SUMMARY

	time	distance	YTD time	YTD distance
swim				
bike				
run				
strength				
other				
total				

notes

_____

_____

_____

_____

_____

_____

_____

period: _____   planned hours: _____

MONDAY _____ / ____ / _____

▨ sleep ▨ fatigue ▨ stress ▨ soreness

resting heart rate _____ weight _____

WORKOUT 1 S B R O _____

planned workout _____

_____

route _____ dist. _____ time _____

avg. HR _____ avg. power _____

zone 1 _____ 2 _____ 3 _____ 4 _____ 5 _____

WORKOUT 2 S B R O _____

planned workout _____

_____

route _____ dist. _____ time _____

avg. HR _____ avg. power _____

zone 1 _____ 2 _____ 3 _____ 4 _____ 5 _____

notes _____

_____

_____

_____

_____

_____

_____

_____

_____

_____

nutrition _____

_____

_____

_____

TUESDAY _____ / ____ / _____

▨ sleep ▨ fatigue ▨ stress ▨ soreness

resting heart rate _____ weight _____

WORKOUT 1 S B R O _____

planned workout _____

_____

route _____ dist. _____ time _____

avg. HR _____ avg. power _____

zone 1 _____ 2 _____ 3 _____ 4 _____ 5 _____

WORKOUT 2 S B R O _____

planned workout _____

_____

route _____ dist. _____ time _____

avg. HR _____ avg. power _____

zone 1 _____ 2 _____ 3 _____ 4 _____ 5 _____

notes _____

_____

_____

_____

_____

_____

_____

_____

_____

nutrition _____

_____

_____

_____

week goals: ▪ _____

▪ _____

▪ _____

WEDNESDAY ____ / ____ / ____

▪ sleep ▪ fatigue ▪ stress ▪ soreness

resting heart rate_____ weight _____

WORKOUT 1 S B R O _____

planned workout _____

_____

route _____ dist. _____ time _____

avg. HR _____ avg. power _____

zone 1____ 2____ 3____ 4____ 5____

WORKOUT 2 S B R O _____

planned workout _____

_____

route _____ dist. _____ time _____

avg. HR _____ avg. power _____

zone 1____ 2____ 3____ 4____ 5____

notes _____

_____

_____

_____

_____

_____

_____

_____

_____

_____

nutrition _____

_____

_____

THURSDAY ____ / ____ / ____

▪ sleep ▪ fatigue ▪ stress ▪ soreness

resting heart rate_____ weight _____

WORKOUT 1 S B R O _____

planned workout _____

_____

route _____ dist. _____ time _____

avg. HR _____ avg. power _____

zone 1____ 2____ 3____ 4____ 5____

WORKOUT 2 S B R O _____

planned workout _____

_____

route _____ dist. _____ time _____

avg. HR _____ avg. power _____

zone 1____ 2____ 3____ 4____ 5____

notes _____

_____

_____

_____

_____

_____

_____

_____

_____

_____

nutrition _____

_____

FRIDAY _____ / ___ / _____

■ sleep ■ fatigue ■ stress ■ soreness

resting heart rate_____ weight _____

WORKOUT 1 S B R O _____

planned workout _____

_____

_____

route _____ dist. _____ time _____

avg. HR _____ avg. power _____

zone 1_____ 2_____ 3_____ 4_____ 5_____

WORKOUT 2 S B R O _____

planned workout _____

_____

route _____ dist. _____ time _____

avg. HR _____ avg. power _____

zone 1_____ 2_____ 3_____ 4_____ 5_____

notes _____

_____

_____

_____

_____

_____

_____

_____

_____

nutrition _____

_____

_____

SATURDAY _____ / ___ / _____

■ sleep ■ fatigue ■ stress ■ soreness

resting heart rate_____ weight _____

WORKOUT 1 S B R O _____

planned workout _____

_____

_____

route _____ dist. _____ time _____

avg. HR _____ avg. power _____

zone 1_____ 2_____ 3_____ 4_____ 5_____

WORKOUT 2 S B R O _____

planned workout _____

_____

route _____ dist. _____ time _____

avg. HR _____ avg. power _____

zone 1_____ 2_____ 3_____ 4_____ 5_____

notes _____

_____

_____

_____

_____

_____

_____

_____

_____

nutrition _____

_____

_____

SUNDAY ___ / ___ / ___

▨ sleep ▨ fatigue ▨ stress ▨ soreness

resting heart rate_____weight _____

WORKOUT 1 S B R O _____

planned workout_____

_____

_____

route _____dist. _____time _____

avg. HR_____avg. power_____

zone 1_____2_____3_____4_____5_____

WORKOUT 2 S B R O _____

planned workout_____

_____

route _____dist. _____time _____

avg. HR_____avg. power_____

zone 1_____2_____3_____4_____5_____

notes _____

_____

_____

_____

_____

_____

_____

_____

_____

_____

_____

nutrition _____

_____

_____

_____

WEEKLY SUMMARY

	time	distance	YTD time	YTD distance
swim				
bike				
run				
strength				
other				
total				

notes

_____

_____

_____

_____

_____

_____

_____

_____

period: _____   planned hours: _____

MONDAY _____ / _____ / _____

▨ sleep ▨ fatigue ▨ stress ▨ soreness

resting heart rate _____ weight _____

WORKOUT 1 S B R O _____

planned workout _____

_____

route _____ dist. _____ time _____

avg. HR _____ avg. power _____

zone 1 _____ 2 _____ 3 _____ 4 _____ 5 _____

WORKOUT 2 S B R O _____

planned workout _____

_____

route _____ dist. _____ time _____

avg. HR _____ avg. power _____

zone 1 _____ 2 _____ 3 _____ 4 _____ 5 _____

notes _____

_____

_____

_____

_____

_____

_____

_____

_____

_____

nutrition _____

_____

_____

_____

TUESDAY _____ / _____ / _____

▨ sleep ▨ fatigue ▨ stress ▨ soreness

resting heart rate _____ weight _____

WORKOUT 1 S B R O _____

planned workout _____

_____

route _____ dist. _____ time _____

avg. HR _____ avg. power _____

zone 1 _____ 2 _____ 3 _____ 4 _____ 5 _____

WORKOUT 2 S B R O _____

planned workout _____

_____

route _____ dist. _____ time _____

avg. HR _____ avg. power _____

zone 1 _____ 2 _____ 3 _____ 4 _____ 5 _____

notes _____

_____

_____

_____

_____

_____

_____

_____

_____

_____

_____

_____

nutrition _____

_____

_____

week goals: ■ _____
■ _____
■ _____

WEDNESDAY _____ / _____ / _____

■ sleep ■ fatigue ■ stress ■ soreness

resting heart rate _____ weight _____

WORKOUT 1 S B R O _____

planned workout _____

_____

route _____ dist. _____ time _____

avg. HR _____ avg. power _____

zone 1 _____ 2 _____ 3 _____ 4 _____ 5 _____

WORKOUT 2 S B R O _____

planned workout _____

_____

route _____ dist. _____ time _____

avg. HR _____ avg. power _____

zone 1 _____ 2 _____ 3 _____ 4 _____ 5 _____

notes _____
_____
_____
_____
_____
_____
_____
_____
_____

nutrition _____
_____
_____
_____
_____

THURSDAY _____ / _____ / _____

■ sleep ■ fatigue ■ stress ■ soreness

resting heart rate _____ weight _____

WORKOUT 1 S B R O _____

planned workout _____

_____

route _____ dist. _____ time _____

avg. HR _____ avg. power _____

zone 1 _____ 2 _____ 3 _____ 4 _____ 5 _____

WORKOUT 2 S B R O _____

planned workout _____

_____

route _____ dist. _____ time _____

avg. HR _____ avg. power _____

zone 1 _____ 2 _____ 3 _____ 4 _____ 5 _____

notes _____
_____
_____
_____
_____
_____
_____
_____
_____

nutrition _____
_____
_____
_____

FRIDAY_____ / ____ /

■ sleep ■ fatigue ■ stress ■ soreness

resting heart rate_____weight _____

WORKOUT 1 S B R O _____

planned workout _____

_____

_____

route _____dist. _____time _____

avg. HR _____avg. power _____

zone 1____ 2____ 3____ 4____ 5____

WORKOUT 2 S B R O _____

planned workout _____

_____

route _____dist. _____time _____

avg. HR _____avg. power _____

zone 1____ 2____ 3____ 4____ 5____

notes _____

_____

_____

_____

_____

_____

_____

_____

_____

nutrition _____

_____

_____

_____

SATURDAY_____ / ____ /

■ sleep ■ fatigue ■ stress ■ soreness

resting heart rate_____ weight _____

WORKOUT 1 S B R O _____

planned workout _____

_____

_____

route _____dist. _____time _____

avg. HR _____avg. power _____

zone 1____ 2____ 3____ 4____ 5____

WORKOUT 2 S B R O _____

planned workout _____

_____

_____

route _____dist. _____time _____

avg. HR _____avg. power _____

zone 1____ 2____ 3____ 4____ 5____

notes _____

_____

_____

_____

_____

_____

_____

_____

_____

nutrition _____

_____

_____

_____

SUNDAY _____ / ___ / _____

☐ sleep ☐ fatigue ☐ stress ☐ soreness

resting heart rate_____ weight _____

WORKOUT 1 S B R O _____

planned workout_____

_____

_____

route _____ dist. _____ time _____

avg. HR_____ avg. power _____

zone 1_____ 2 _____ 3_____ 4_____ 5_____

WORKOUT 2 S B R O _____

planned workout_____

_____

route _____ dist. _____ time _____

avg. HR_____ avg. power _____

zone 1_____ 2 _____ 3_____ 4_____ 5_____

notes _____

_____

_____

_____

_____

_____

_____

_____

_____

_____

_____

_____

nutrition _____

_____

_____

_____

WEEKLY SUMMARY

	time	distance	YTD time	YTD distance
swim				
bike				
run				
strength				
other				
total				

notes

_____

_____

_____

_____

_____

_____

_____

_____

week beginning: _____

period: _____   planned hours: _____

MONDAY _____ / _____ /

■ sleep ■ fatigue ■ stress ■ soreness

resting heart rate_____ weight _____

WORKOUT 1 S B R O _____

planned workout _____

_____

route _____ dist. _____ time _____

avg. HR _____ avg. power _____

zone 1____ 2____ 3____ 4____ 5____

WORKOUT 2 S B R O _____

planned workout _____

_____

route _____ dist. _____ time _____

avg. HR _____ avg. power _____

zone 1____ 2____ 3____ 4____ 5____

notes _____

_____

_____

_____

_____

_____

_____

_____

_____

_____

nutrition _____

_____

_____

_____

TUESDAY _____ / _____ /

■ sleep ■ fatigue ■ stress ■ soreness

resting heart rate_____ weight _____

WORKOUT 1 S B R O _____

planned workout _____

_____

route _____ dist. _____ time _____

avg. HR _____ avg. power _____

zone 1____ 2____ 3____ 4____ 5____

WORKOUT 2 S B R O _____

planned workout _____

_____

route _____ dist. _____ time _____

avg. HR _____ avg. power _____

zone 1____ 2____ 3____ 4____ 5____

notes _____

_____

_____

_____

_____

_____

_____

_____

_____

nutrition _____

_____

_____

week goals: ▦ _____

▦ _____

▦ _____

WEDNESDAY ____ / ____ / ____

▦ sleep ▦ fatigue ▦ stress ▦ soreness

resting heart rate _____ weight _____

WORKOUT 1 S B R O _____

planned workout _____

_____

route _____ dist. _____ time _____

avg. HR _____ avg. power _____

zone 1 ____ 2 ____ 3 ____ 4 ____ 5 ____

WORKOUT 2 S B R O _____

planned workout _____

_____

route _____ dist. _____ time _____

avg. HR _____ avg. power _____

zone 1 ____ 2 ____ 3 ____ 4 ____ 5 ____

notes _____

_____

_____

_____

_____

_____

_____

_____

_____

nutrition _____

_____

_____

_____

THURSDAY ____ / ____ / ____

▦ sleep ▦ fatigue ▦ stress ▦ soreness

resting heart rate _____ weight _____

WORKOUT 1 S B R O _____

planned workout _____

_____

route _____ dist. _____ time _____

avg. HR _____ avg. power _____

zone 1 ____ 2 ____ 3 ____ 4 ____ 5 ____

WORKOUT 2 S B R O _____

planned workout _____

_____

route _____ dist. _____ time _____

avg. HR _____ avg. power _____

zone 1 ____ 2 ____ 3 ____ 4 ____ 5 ____

notes _____

_____

_____

_____

_____

_____

_____

_____

_____

nutrition _____

_____

_____

_____

FRIDAY _____ / _____ / _____

sleep ▨ fatigue ▨ stress ▨ soreness ▨

resting heart rate _____ weight _____

WORKOUT 1 S B R O _____

planned workout _____

_____

_____

route _____ dist. _____ time _____

avg. HR _____ avg. power _____

zone 1 _____ 2 _____ 3 _____ 4 _____ 5 _____

WORKOUT 2 S B R O _____

planned workout _____

_____

route _____ dist. _____ time _____

avg. HR _____ avg. power _____

zone 1 _____ 2 _____ 3 _____ 4 _____ 5 _____

notes _____

_____

_____

_____

_____

_____

_____

_____

_____

_____

_____

_____

nutrition _____

_____

_____

_____

SATURDAY _____ / _____ / _____

sleep ▨ fatigue ▨ stress ▨ soreness ▨

resting heart rate _____ weight _____

WORKOUT 1 S B R O _____

planned workout _____

_____

_____

route _____ dist. _____ time _____

avg. HR _____ avg. power _____

zone 1 _____ 2 _____ 3 _____ 4 _____ 5 _____

WORKOUT 2 S B R O _____

planned workout _____

_____

_____

route _____ dist. _____ time _____

avg. HR _____ avg. power _____

zone 1 _____ 2 _____ 3 _____ 4 _____ 5 _____

notes _____

_____

_____

_____

_____

_____

_____

_____

_____

_____

_____

_____

nutrition _____

_____

_____

SUNDAY ____ / ____ / ____

■ sleep ■ fatigue ■ stress ■ soreness

resting heart rate_____ weight _____

WORKOUT 1 S B R O _____

planned workout_____

_____

_____

route _____ dist. _____ time _____

avg. HR _____ avg. power _____

zone 1_____ 2_____ 3_____ 4_____ 5_____

WORKOUT 2 S B R O _____

planned workout_____

_____

route _____ dist. _____ time _____

avg. HR _____ avg. power _____

zone 1_____ 2_____ 3_____ 4_____ 5_____

notes _____

_____

_____

_____

_____

_____

_____

_____

_____

_____

nutrition _____

_____

_____

_____

WEEKLY SUMMARY

	time	distance	YTD time	YTD distance
swim				
bike				
run				
strength				
other				
total				

notes

_____

_____

_____

_____

_____

_____

_____

period: _____   planned hours: _____

MONDAY _____ / _____ / _____   **notes** _____

◻ sleep ◻ fatigue ◻ stress ◻ soreness   _____

resting heart rate_____ weight _____   _____

WORKOUT 1 S B R O _____   _____

planned workout _____   _____

_____   _____

route _____ dist. _____ time _____   _____

avg. HR_____ avg. power _____   _____

zone 1_____ 2_____ 3_____ 4_____ 5_____   _____

WORKOUT 2 S B R O _____   _____

planned workout _____   _____

_____   **nutrition** _____

route _____ dist. _____ time _____   _____

avg. HR_____ avg. power _____   _____

zone 1_____ 2_____ 3_____ 4_____ 5_____   _____

TUESDAY _____ / _____ / _____   **notes** _____

◻ sleep ◻ fatigue ◻ stress ◻ soreness   _____

resting heart rate_____ weight _____   _____

WORKOUT 1 S B R O _____   _____

planned workout _____   _____

_____   _____

route _____ dist. _____ time _____   _____

avg. HR_____ avg. power _____   _____

zone 1_____ 2_____ 3_____ 4_____ 5_____   _____

WORKOUT 2 S B R O _____   _____

planned workout _____   _____

_____   **nutrition** _____

route _____ dist. _____ time _____   _____

avg. HR_____ avg. power _____   _____

zone 1_____ 2_____ 3_____ 4_____ 5_____   _____

week goals: ▪ _____

▪ _____

▪ _____

WEDNESDAY ____ / ____ / ____

▪ sleep ▪ fatigue ▪ stress ▪ soreness

resting heart rate_____ weight _____

WORKOUT 1 S B R O _____

planned workout _____

_____

route _____ dist. _____ time _____

avg. HR _____ avg. power _____

zone 1____ 2_____ 3_____ 4_____ 5_____

WORKOUT 2 S B R O _____

planned workout _____

_____

route _____ dist. _____ time _____

avg. HR _____ avg. power _____

zone 1____ 2_____ 3_____ 4_____ 5_____

notes _____

_____

_____

_____

_____

_____

_____

_____

_____

_____

nutrition _____

_____

_____

_____

THURSDAY ____ / ____ / ____

▪ sleep ▪ fatigue ▪ stress ▪ soreness

resting heart rate_____ weight _____

WORKOUT 1 S B R O _____

planned workout _____

_____

route _____ dist. _____ time _____

avg. HR _____ avg. power _____

zone 1____ 2_____ 3_____ 4_____ 5_____

WORKOUT 2 S B R O _____

planned workout _____

_____

route _____ dist. _____ time _____

avg. HR _____ avg. power _____

zone 1____ 2_____ 3_____ 4_____ 5_____

notes _____

_____

_____

_____

_____

_____

_____

_____

_____

nutrition _____

_____

_____

_____

FRIDAY ___ / ___ / ___

▨ sleep ▨ fatigue ▨ stress ▨ soreness

resting heart rate_____ weight _____

WORKOUT 1 S B R O _____

planned workout _____

_____

_____

route _____ dist. _____ time _____

avg. HR _____ avg. power _____

zone 1____ 2____ 3____ 4____ 5____

WORKOUT 2 S B R O _____

planned workout _____

_____

route _____ dist. _____ time _____

avg. HR _____ avg. power _____

zone 1____ 2____ 3____ 4____ 5____

notes _____

_____

_____

_____

_____

_____

_____

_____

_____

nutrition _____

_____

_____

SATURDAY ___ / ___ / ___

▨ sleep ▨ fatigue ▨ stress ▨ soreness

resting heart rate_____ weight _____

WORKOUT 1 S B R O _____

planned workout _____

_____

_____

route _____ dist. _____ time _____

avg. HR _____ avg. power _____

zone 1____ 2____ 3____ 4____ 5____

WORKOUT 2 S B R O _____

planned workout _____

_____

route _____ dist. _____ time _____

avg. HR _____ avg. power _____

zone 1____ 2____ 3____ 4____ 5____

notes _____

_____

_____

_____

_____

_____

_____

_____

_____

_____

nutrition _____

_____

SUNDAY ___ / ___ / ___

☐ sleep ☐ fatigue ☐ stress ☐ soreness

resting heart rate_____ weight _____

WORKOUT 1 S B R O _____

planned workout _____

_____

_____

route _____ dist. _____ time _____

avg. HR _____ avg. power _____

zone 1_____ 2_____ 3_____ 4_____ 5_____

WORKOUT 2 S B R O _____

planned workout _____

_____

route _____ dist. _____ time _____

avg. HR _____ avg. power _____

zone 1_____ 2_____ 3_____ 4_____ 5_____

notes _____

_____

_____

_____

_____

_____

_____

_____

nutrition _____

_____

_____

_____

WEEKLY SUMMARY

	time	distance	YTD time	YTD distance
swim				
bike				
run				
strength				
other				
total				

notes

_____

_____

_____

_____

_____

_____

_____

week beginning: _____

period: _____   planned hours: _____

MONDAY _____ / _____ / _____

▨ sleep ▨ fatigue ▨ stress ▨ soreness

resting heart rate _____ weight _____

WORKOUT 1   S   B   R   O _____

planned workout _____

_____

route _____ dist. _____ time _____

avg. HR _____ avg. power _____

zone 1_____ 2_____ 3_____ 4_____ 5_____

WORKOUT 2   S   B   R   O _____

planned workout _____

_____

route _____ dist. _____ time _____

avg. HR _____ avg. power _____

zone 1_____ 2_____ 3_____ 4_____ 5_____

notes _____

_____

_____

_____

_____

_____

_____

_____

_____

_____

_____

nutrition _____

_____

_____

_____

TUESDAY _____ / _____ / _____

▨ sleep ▨ fatigue ▨ stress ▨ soreness

resting heart rate _____ weight _____

WORKOUT 1   S   B   R   O _____

planned workout _____

_____

route _____ dist. _____ time _____

avg. HR _____ avg. power _____

zone 1_____ 2_____ 3_____ 4_____ 5_____

WORKOUT 2   S   B   R   O _____

planned workout _____

_____

route _____ dist. _____ time _____

avg. HR _____ avg. power _____

zone 1_____ 2_____ 3_____ 4_____ 5_____

notes _____

_____

_____

_____

_____

_____

_____

_____

_____

_____

nutrition _____

_____

_____

_____

week goals: ▪ _____

▪ _____

▪ _____

WEDNESDAY ____ / ____ / ____

▪ sleep ▪ fatigue ▪ stress ▪ soreness

resting heart rate_____ weight _____

WORKOUT 1 S B R O _____

planned workout_____

_____

route _____ dist. _____ time _____

avg. HR _____ avg. power _____

zone 1____ 2____ 3____ 4____ 5____

WORKOUT 2 S B R O _____

planned workout_____

_____

route _____ dist. _____ time _____

avg. HR _____ avg. power _____

zone 1____ 2____ 3____ 4____ 5____

notes _____

_____

_____

_____

_____

_____

_____

_____

_____

nutrition _____

_____

_____

_____

THURSDAY ____ / ____ / ____

▪ sleep ▪ fatigue ▪ stress ▪ soreness

resting heart rate_____ weight _____

WORKOUT 1 S B R O _____

planned workout_____

_____

route _____ dist. _____ time _____

avg. HR _____ avg. power _____

zone 1____ 2____ 3____ 4____ 5____

WORKOUT 2 S B R O _____

planned workout_____

_____

route _____ dist. _____ time _____

avg. HR _____ avg. power _____

zone 1____ 2____ 3____ 4____ 5____

notes _____

_____

_____

_____

_____

_____

_____

_____

_____

nutrition _____

_____

_____

_____

FRIDAY ___ / ___ / ___

▨ sleep ▨ fatigue ▨ stress ▨ soreness

resting heart rate_____ weight _____

WORKOUT 1 S B R O _____

planned workout _____

_____

_____

route _____ dist. _____ time _____

avg. HR_____ avg. power_____

zone 1_____ 2_____ 3_____ 4_____ 5_____

WORKOUT 2 S B R O _____

planned workout _____

_____

route _____ dist. _____ time _____

avg. HR_____ avg. power_____

zone 1_____ 2_____ 3_____ 4_____ 5_____

notes _____

_____

_____

_____

_____

_____

_____

_____

_____

_____

_____

_____

nutrition _____

_____

_____

_____

SATURDAY ___ / ___ / ___

▨ sleep ▨ fatigue ▨ stress ▨ soreness

resting heart rate_____ weight _____

WORKOUT 1 S B R O _____

planned workout _____

_____

_____

route _____ dist. _____ time _____

avg. HR_____ avg. power_____

zone 1_____ 2_____ 3_____ 4_____ 5_____

WORKOUT 2 S B R O _____

planned workout _____

_____

_____

route _____ dist. _____ time _____

avg. HR_____ avg. power_____

zone 1_____ 2_____ 3_____ 4_____ 5_____

notes _____

_____

_____

_____

_____

_____

_____

_____

_____

_____

nutrition _____

_____

_____

SUNDAY _____ / ___ / _____

☐ sleep ☐ fatigue ☐ stress ☐ soreness

resting heart rate_____ weight _____

WORKOUT 1 S B R O _____

planned workout_____

_____

_____

route_____ dist. _____ time _____

avg. HR_____ avg. power_____

zone 1_____ 2_____ 3_____ 4_____ 5_____

WORKOUT 2 S B R O _____

planned workout_____

_____

route_____ dist. _____ time _____

avg. HR_____ avg. power_____

zone 1_____ 2_____ 3_____ 4_____ 5_____

notes _____

_____

_____

_____

_____

_____

_____

_____

_____

_____

_____

nutrition _____

_____

_____

_____

WEEKLY SUMMARY

	time	distance	YTD time	YTD distance
swim				
bike				
run				
strength				
other				
total				

notes

_____

_____

_____

_____

_____

_____

_____

_____

period: _____   planned hours: _____

MONDAY _____ / ____ / _____

▭ sleep ▭ fatigue ▭ stress ▭ soreness

resting heart rate_____ weight _____

WORKOUT 1 S B R O _____

planned workout_____

_____

route _____dist. _____time _____

avg. HR_____avg. power_____

zone 1_____2_____3_____4_____5_____

WORKOUT 2 S B R O _____

planned workout_____

_____

route _____dist. _____time _____

avg. HR_____avg. power_____

zone 1_____2_____3_____4_____5_____

notes _____

_____

_____

_____

_____

_____

_____

_____

_____

_____

_____

nutrition _____

_____

_____

_____

TUESDAY _____ / ____ / _____

▭ sleep ▭ fatigue ▭ stress ▭ soreness

resting heart rate_____ weight _____

WORKOUT 1 S B R O _____

planned workout_____

_____

route _____dist. _____time _____

avg. HR_____avg. power_____

zone 1_____2_____3_____4_____5_____

WORKOUT 2 S B R O _____

planned workout_____

_____

route _____dist. _____time _____

avg. HR_____avg. power_____

zone 1_____2_____3_____4_____5_____

notes _____

_____

_____

_____

_____

_____

_____

_____

_____

nutrition _____

_____

_____

week goals: ▦ _____
▦ _____
▦ _____

WEDNESDAY ____ / ____ / ____

▦ sleep ▦ fatigue ▦ stress ▦ soreness

resting heart rate_____ weight _____

WORKOUT 1 S B R O _____

planned workout _____
_____

route _____ dist. _____ time _____

avg. HR _____ avg. power _____

zone 1_____ 2_____ 3_____ 4_____ 5_____

WORKOUT 2 S B R O _____

planned workout _____
_____

route _____ dist. _____ time _____

avg. HR _____ avg. power _____

zone 1_____ 2_____ 3_____ 4_____ 5_____

notes _____
_____
_____
_____
_____
_____
_____
_____
_____

nutrition _____
_____
_____
_____

THURSDAY ____ / ____ / ____

▦ sleep ▦ fatigue ▦ stress ▦ soreness

resting heart rate_____ weight _____

WORKOUT 1 S B R O _____

planned workout _____
_____

route _____ dist. _____ time _____

avg. HR _____ avg. power _____

zone 1_____ 2_____ 3_____ 4_____ 5_____

WORKOUT 2 S B R O _____

planned workout _____
_____

route _____ dist. _____ time _____

avg. HR _____ avg. power _____

zone 1_____ 2_____ 3_____ 4_____ 5_____

notes _____
_____
_____
_____
_____
_____
_____
_____
_____

nutrition _____
_____
_____
_____

FRIDAY ___ / ___ / ___

▨ sleep ▨ fatigue ▨ stress ▨ soreness

resting heart rate _____ weight _____

WORKOUT 1 S B R O _____

planned workout _____

_____

_____

route _____ dist. _____ time _____

avg. HR _____ avg. power _____

zone 1 _____ 2 _____ 3 _____ 4 _____ 5 _____

WORKOUT 2 S B R O _____

planned workout _____

_____

route _____ dist. _____ time _____

avg. HR _____ avg. power _____

zone 1 _____ 2 _____ 3 _____ 4 _____ 5 _____

notes _____

_____

_____

_____

_____

_____

_____

_____

_____

_____

_____

nutrition _____

_____

_____

SATURDAY ___ / ___ / ___

▨ sleep ▨ fatigue ▨ stress ▨ soreness

resting heart rate _____ weight _____

WORKOUT 1 S B R O _____

planned workout _____

_____

_____

route _____ dist. _____ time _____

avg. HR _____ avg. power _____

zone 1 _____ 2 _____ 3 _____ 4 _____ 5 _____

WORKOUT 2 S B R O _____

planned workout _____

_____

_____

route _____ dist. _____ time _____

avg. HR _____ avg. power _____

zone 1 _____ 2 _____ 3 _____ 4 _____ 5 _____

notes _____

_____

_____

_____

_____

_____

_____

_____

_____

_____

_____

nutrition _____

_____

_____

SUNDAY ___ / ___ / ___

■ sleep ■ fatigue ■ stress ■ soreness

resting heart rate_____ weight _____

WORKOUT 1 S B R O _____

planned workout_____

_____

_____

route _____ dist. _____ time _____

avg. HR _____ avg. power _____

zone 1____ 2____ 3____ 4____ 5____

WORKOUT 2 S B R O _____

planned workout_____

_____

route _____ dist. _____ time _____

avg. HR _____ avg. power _____

zone 1____ 2____ 3____ 4____ 5____

notes _____

_____

_____

_____

_____

_____

_____

_____

_____

_____

_____

_____

nutrition _____

_____

_____

_____

WEEKLY SUMMARY

	time	distance	YTD time	YTD distance
swim				
bike				
run				
strength				
other				
total				

notes

_____

_____

_____

_____

_____

_____

_____

_____

period: _____   planned hours: _____

MONDAY _____ / _____ / _____

▨ sleep ▨ fatigue ▨ stress ▨ soreness

resting heart rate_____ weight _____

WORKOUT 1 S B R O _____

planned workout _____

_____

route _____ dist. _____ time _____

avg. HR _____ avg. power _____

zone 1____ 2____ 3____ 4____ 5____

WORKOUT 2 S B R O _____

planned workout _____

_____

route _____ dist. _____ time _____

avg. HR _____ avg. power _____

zone 1____ 2____ 3____ 4____ 5____

notes _____

_____

_____

_____

_____

_____

_____

_____

_____

_____

_____

_____

nutrition _____

_____

_____

_____

TUESDAY _____ / _____ / _____

▨ sleep ▨ fatigue ▨ stress ▨ soreness

resting heart rate_____ weight _____

WORKOUT 1 S B R O _____

planned workout _____

_____

route _____ dist. _____ time _____

avg. HR _____ avg. power _____

zone 1____ 2____ 3____ 4____ 5____

WORKOUT 2 S B R O _____

planned workout _____

_____

route _____ dist. _____ time _____

avg. HR _____ avg. power _____

zone 1____ 2____ 3____ 4____ 5____

notes _____

_____

_____

_____

_____

_____

_____

_____

_____

_____

_____

nutrition _____

_____

_____

week goals: ■ _____

■ _____

■ _____

WEDNESDAY ____ / ____ / ____

■ sleep ■ fatigue ■ stress ■ soreness

resting heart rate_____ weight _____

WORKOUT 1 S B R O _____

planned workout_____

_____

route _____dist. _____time _____

avg. HR_____avg. power_____

zone 1_____ 2_____ 3_____ 4_____ 5_____

WORKOUT 2 S B R O _____

planned workout_____

_____

route _____dist. _____time _____

avg. HR_____avg. power_____

zone 1_____ 2_____ 3_____ 4_____ 5_____

notes _____

_____

_____

_____

_____

_____

_____

_____

_____

_____

nutrition _____

_____

_____

_____

THURSDAY ____ / ____ / ____

■ sleep ■ fatigue ■ stress ■ soreness

resting heart rate_____ weight _____

WORKOUT 1 S B R O _____

planned workout_____

_____

route _____dist. _____time _____

avg. HR_____avg. power_____

zone 1_____ 2_____ 3_____ 4_____ 5_____

WORKOUT 2 S B R O _____

planned workout_____

_____

route _____dist. _____time _____

avg. HR_____avg. power_____

zone 1_____ 2_____ 3_____ 4_____ 5_____

notes _____

_____

_____

_____

_____

_____

_____

_____

nutrition _____

_____

_____

FRIDAY _____ / ____ / ____

☐ sleep ☐ fatigue ☐ stress ☐ soreness

resting heart rate _____ weight _____

WORKOUT 1 S B R O _____

planned workout _____

_____

_____

route _____ dist. _____ time _____

avg. HR _____ avg. power _____

zone 1 _____ 2 _____ 3 _____ 4 _____ 5 _____

WORKOUT 2 S B R O _____

planned workout _____

_____

route _____ dist. _____ time _____

avg. HR _____ avg. power _____

zone 1 _____ 2 _____ 3 _____ 4 _____ 5 _____

notes _____

_____

_____

_____

_____

_____

_____

_____

_____

nutrition _____

_____

_____

_____

SATURDAY _____ / ____ / ____

☐ sleep ☐ fatigue ☐ stress ☐ soreness

resting heart rate _____ weight _____

WORKOUT 1 S B R O _____

planned workout _____

_____

_____

route _____ dist. _____ time _____

avg. HR _____ avg. power _____

zone 1 _____ 2 _____ 3 _____ 4 _____ 5 _____

WORKOUT 2 S B R O _____

planned workout _____

_____

_____

route _____ dist. _____ time _____

avg. HR _____ avg. power _____

zone 1 _____ 2 _____ 3 _____ 4 _____ 5 _____

notes _____

_____

_____

_____

_____

_____

_____

_____

_____

nutrition _____

_____

_____

_____

SUNDAY _____ / ___ / _____

▨ sleep ▨ fatigue ▨ stress ▨ soreness

resting heart rate_____ weight _____

WORKOUT 1 S B R O _____

planned workout _____

_____

_____

route _____ dist. _____ time _____

avg. HR _____ avg. power _____

zone 1_____ 2 _____ 3 _____ 4 _____ 5 _____

WORKOUT 2 S B R O _____

planned workout _____

_____

route _____ dist. _____ time _____

avg. HR _____ avg. power _____

zone 1_____ 2 _____ 3 _____ 4 _____ 5 _____

notes _____

_____

_____

_____

_____

_____

_____

_____

_____

_____

nutrition _____

_____

_____

_____

WEEKLY SUMMARY

	time	distance	YTD time	YTD distance
swim				
bike				
run				
strength				
other				
total				

notes

_____

_____

_____

_____

_____

_____

_____

_____

period: _____   planned hours: _____

MONDAY _____ / ____ / _____   notes _____

▒ sleep ▒ fatigue ▒ stress ▒ soreness   _____

resting heart rate_____ weight _____   _____

WORKOUT 1 S B R O _____   _____

planned workout_____   _____

_____   _____

route _____ dist. _____ time _____   _____

avg. HR_____ avg. power _____   _____

zone 1_____ 2_____ 3_____ 4_____ 5_____   _____

WORKOUT 2 S B R O _____   _____

planned workout_____   _____

_____   **nutrition** _____

route _____ dist. _____ time _____   _____

avg. HR_____ avg. power _____   _____

zone 1_____ 2_____ 3_____ 4_____ 5_____   _____

TUESDAY _____ / ____ / _____   notes _____

▒ sleep ▒ fatigue ▒ stress ▒ soreness   _____

resting heart rate_____ weight _____   _____

WORKOUT 1 S B R O _____   _____

planned workout_____   _____

_____   _____

route _____ dist. _____ time _____   _____

avg. HR_____ avg. power _____   _____

zone 1_____ 2_____ 3_____ 4_____ 5_____   _____

WORKOUT 2 S B R O _____   _____

planned workout_____   _____

_____   **nutrition** _____

route _____ dist. _____ time _____   _____

avg. HR_____ avg. power _____   _____

zone 1_____ 2_____ 3_____ 4_____ 5_____   _____

week goals: ▪ _____
▪ _____
▪ _____

WEDNESDAY ____ / ____ / ____

▪ sleep ▪ fatigue ▪ stress ▪ soreness

resting heart rate_____ weight _____

WORKOUT 1 S B R O _____

planned workout _____

_____

route _____ dist. _____ time _____

avg. HR _____ avg. power _____

zone 1_____ 2_____ 3_____ 4_____ 5_____

WORKOUT 2 S B R O _____

planned workout _____

_____

route _____ dist. _____ time _____

avg. HR _____ avg. power _____

zone 1_____ 2_____ 3_____ 4_____ 5_____

notes _____
_____
_____
_____
_____
_____
_____
_____
_____

nutrition _____
_____

THURSDAY ____ / ____ / ____

▪ sleep ▪ fatigue ▪ stress ▪ soreness

resting heart rate_____ weight _____

WORKOUT 1 S B R O _____

planned workout _____

_____

route _____ dist. _____ time _____

avg. HR _____ avg. power _____

zone 1_____ 2_____ 3_____ 4_____ 5_____

WORKOUT 2 S B R O _____

planned workout _____

_____

route _____ dist. _____ time _____

avg. HR _____ avg. power _____

zone 1_____ 2_____ 3_____ 4_____ 5_____

notes _____
_____
_____
_____
_____
_____
_____
_____
_____

nutrition _____
_____

FRIDAY _____ / / _____

◻ sleep ◻ fatigue ◻ stress ◻ soreness

resting heart rate_____ weight _____

WORKOUT 1 S B R O _____

planned workout _____

_____

_____

route _____ dist. _____ time _____

avg. HR _____ avg. power _____

zone 1____ 2____ 3____ 4____ 5____

WORKOUT 2 S B R O _____

planned workout _____

_____

route _____ dist. _____ time _____

avg. HR _____ avg. power _____

zone 1____ 2____ 3____ 4____ 5____

notes _____

_____

_____

_____

_____

_____

_____

_____

_____

_____

_____

nutrition _____

_____

_____

_____

SATURDAY _____ / / _____

◻ sleep ◻ fatigue ◻ stress ◻ soreness

resting heart rate_____ weight _____

WORKOUT 1 S B R O _____

planned workout _____

_____

_____

route _____ dist. _____ time _____

avg. HR _____ avg. power _____

zone 1____ 2____ 3____ 4____ 5____

WORKOUT 2 S B R O _____

planned workout _____

_____

_____

route _____ dist. _____ time _____

avg. HR _____ avg. power _____

zone 1____ 2____ 3____ 4____ 5____

notes _____

_____

_____

_____

_____

_____

_____

_____

_____

_____

nutrition _____

_____

_____

_____

SUNDAY _____ / _____ / _____

☐ sleep ☐ fatigue ☐ stress ☐ soreness

resting heart rate_____ weight _____

WORKOUT 1 S B R O _____

planned workout _____

_____

_____

route _____ dist. _____ time _____

avg. HR_____ avg. power _____

zone 1_____ 2_____ 3_____ 4_____ 5_____

WORKOUT 2 S B R O _____

planned workout _____

_____

route _____ dist. _____ time _____

avg. HR_____ avg. power _____

zone 1_____ 2_____ 3_____ 4_____ 5_____

notes _____

_____

_____

_____

_____

_____

_____

_____

_____

_____

_____

nutrition _____

_____

_____

WEEKLY SUMMARY

	time	distance	YTD time	YTD distance
swim				
bike				
run				
strength				
other				
total				

notes

_____

_____

_____

_____

_____

_____

_____

_____

period: _____   planned hours: _____

MONDAY _____ / ____ / _____

☐ sleep ☐ fatigue ☐ stress ☐ soreness

resting heart rate_____ weight _____

WORKOUT 1 S B R O _____

planned workout _____

_____

route _____ dist. _____ time _____

avg. HR _____ avg. power _____

zone 1_____ 2_____ 3_____ 4_____ 5_____

WORKOUT 2 S B R O _____

planned workout _____

_____

route _____ dist. _____ time _____

avg. HR _____ avg. power _____

zone 1_____ 2_____ 3_____ 4_____ 5_____

notes _____

_____

_____

_____

_____

_____

_____

_____

_____

_____

nutrition _____

_____

_____

_____

TUESDAY _____ / ____ / _____

☐ sleep ☐ fatigue ☐ stress ☐ soreness

resting heart rate_____ weight _____

WORKOUT 1 S B R O _____

planned workout _____

_____

route _____ dist. _____ time _____

avg. HR _____ avg. power _____

zone 1_____ 2_____ 3_____ 4_____ 5_____

WORKOUT 2 S B R O _____

planned workout _____

_____

route _____ dist. _____ time _____

avg. HR _____ avg. power _____

zone 1_____ 2_____ 3_____ 4_____ 5_____

notes _____

_____

_____

_____

_____

_____

_____

_____

_____

_____

nutrition _____

_____

_____

week goals: ■ _____

■ _____

■ _____

WEDNESDAY ____ / ____ / ____

■ sleep ■ fatigue ■ stress ■ soreness

resting heart rate_____ weight _____

WORKOUT 1 S B R O _____

planned workout _____

_____

route _____ dist. _____ time _____

avg. HR _____ avg. power _____

zone 1____ 2____ 3____ 4____ 5____

WORKOUT 2 S B R O _____

planned workout _____

_____

route _____ dist. _____ time _____

avg. HR _____ avg. power _____

zone 1____ 2____ 3____ 4____ 5____

notes _____

_____

_____

_____

_____

_____

_____

_____

_____

nutrition _____

_____

_____

_____

THURSDAY ____ / ____ / ____

■ sleep ■ fatigue ■ stress ■ soreness

resting heart rate_____ weight _____

WORKOUT 1 S B R O _____

planned workout _____

_____

route _____ dist. _____ time _____

avg. HR _____ avg. power _____

zone 1____ 2____ 3____ 4____ 5____

WORKOUT 2 S B R O _____

planned workout _____

_____

route _____ dist. _____ time _____

avg. HR _____ avg. power _____

zone 1____ 2____ 3____ 4____ 5____

notes _____

_____

_____

_____

_____

_____

_____

_____

nutrition _____

_____

_____

_____

FRIDAY ___ / ___ / ___

◻ sleep ◻ fatigue ◻ stress ◻ soreness

resting heart rate_____ weight _____

WORKOUT 1 S B R O _____

planned workout _____

_____

_____

route _____ dist. _____ time _____

avg. HR _____ avg. power _____

zone 1_____ 2_____ 3_____ 4_____ 5_____

WORKOUT 2 S B R O _____

planned workout _____

_____

route _____ dist. _____ time _____

avg. HR _____ avg. power _____

zone 1_____ 2_____ 3_____ 4_____ 5_____

notes _____

_____

_____

_____

_____

_____

_____

_____

_____

_____

_____

_____

nutrition _____

_____

_____

_____

SATURDAY ___ / ___ / ___

◻ sleep ◻ fatigue ◻ stress ◻ soreness

resting heart rate_____ weight _____

WORKOUT 1 S B R O _____

planned workout _____

_____

_____

route _____ dist. _____ time _____

avg. HR _____ avg. power _____

zone 1_____ 2_____ 3_____ 4_____ 5_____

WORKOUT 2 S B R O _____

planned workout _____

_____

_____

route _____ dist. _____ time _____

avg. HR _____ avg. power _____

zone 1_____ 2_____ 3_____ 4_____ 5_____

notes _____

_____

_____

_____

_____

_____

_____

_____

_____

nutrition _____

_____

_____

SUNDAY ___ / ___ / ___

▢ sleep ▢ fatigue ▢ stress ▢ soreness

resting heart rate_____ weight _____

WORKOUT 1 S B R O _____

planned workout_____

_____

_____

route _____dist. _____time _____

avg. HR_____avg. power_____

zone 1_____ 2_____ 3_____ 4_____ 5_____

WORKOUT 2 S B R O _____

planned workout_____

_____

route _____dist. _____time _____

avg. HR_____avg. power_____

zone 1_____ 2_____ 3_____ 4_____ 5_____

notes _____

_____

_____

_____

_____

_____

_____

_____

_____

_____

_____

_____

nutrition _____

_____

_____

_____

WEEKLY SUMMARY

	time	distance	YTD time	YTD distance
swim				
bike				
run				
strength				
other				
total				

notes

_____

_____

_____

_____

_____

_____

_____

_____

period: _____ planned hours: _____

MONDAY _____ / ____ / _____   **notes** _____

▓ sleep ▓ fatigue ▓ stress ▓ soreness   _____

resting heart rate_____ weight _____   _____

WORKOUT 1 S B R O _____   _____

planned workout_____   _____

_____   _____

route _____ dist. _____ time _____   _____

avg. HR_____ avg. power _____   _____

zone 1_____ 2 _____ 3_____ 4_____ 5_____   _____

WORKOUT 2 S B R O _____   _____

planned workout_____   _____

_____   **nutrition** _____

route _____ dist. _____ time _____   _____

avg. HR_____ avg. power _____   _____

zone 1_____ 2 _____ 3_____ 4_____ 5_____   _____

TUESDAY _____ / ____ / _____   **notes** _____

▓ sleep ▓ fatigue ▓ stress ▓ soreness   _____

resting heart rate_____ weight _____   _____

WORKOUT 1 S B R O _____   _____

planned workout_____   _____

_____   _____

route _____ dist. _____ time _____   _____

avg. HR_____ avg. power _____   _____

zone 1_____ 2 _____ 3_____ 4_____ 5_____   _____

WORKOUT 2 S B R O _____   _____

planned workout_____   _____

_____   **nutrition** _____

route _____ dist. _____ time _____   _____

avg. HR_____ avg. power _____   _____

zone 1_____ 2 _____ 3_____ 4_____ 5_____   _____

week goals: ▪ _____

▪ _____

▪ _____

WEDNESDAY ___ / ___ / ___

▪ sleep ▪ fatigue ▪ stress ▪ soreness

resting heart rate_____ weight _____

WORKOUT 1 S B R O _____

planned workout _____

_____

route _____ dist. _____ time _____

avg. HR _____ avg. power _____

zone 1_____ 2_____ 3_____ 4_____ 5_____

WORKOUT 2 S B R O _____

planned workout _____

_____

route _____ dist. _____ time _____

avg. HR _____ avg. power _____

zone 1_____ 2_____ 3_____ 4_____ 5_____

notes _____

_____

_____

_____

_____

_____

_____

_____

_____

_____

_____

nutrition _____

_____

_____

_____

THURSDAY ___ / ___ / ___

▪ sleep ▪ fatigue ▪ stress ▪ soreness

resting heart rate_____ weight _____

WORKOUT 1 S B R O _____

planned workout _____

_____

route _____ dist. _____ time _____

avg. HR _____ avg. power _____

zone 1_____ 2_____ 3_____ 4_____ 5_____

WORKOUT 2 S B R O _____

planned workout _____

_____

route _____ dist. _____ time _____

avg. HR _____ avg. power _____

zone 1_____ 2_____ 3_____ 4_____ 5_____

notes _____

_____

_____

_____

_____

_____

_____

_____

_____

_____

nutrition _____

_____

_____

_____

FRIDAY ____ / ____ / ____

☐ sleep ☐ fatigue ☐ stress ☐ soreness

resting heart rate _____ weight _____

WORKOUT 1 S B R O _____

planned workout _____

_____

_____

route _____ dist. _____ time _____

avg. HR _____ avg. power _____

zone 1____ 2____ 3____ 4____ 5____

WORKOUT 2 S B R O _____

planned workout _____

_____

route _____ dist. _____ time _____

avg. HR _____ avg. power _____

zone 1____ 2____ 3____ 4____ 5____

notes _____

_____

_____

_____

_____

_____

_____

_____

_____

_____

nutrition _____

_____

_____

_____

SATURDAY ____ / ____ / ____

☐ sleep ☐ fatigue ☐ stress ☐ soreness

resting heart rate _____ weight _____

WORKOUT 1 S B R O _____

planned workout _____

_____

_____

route _____ dist. _____ time _____

avg. HR _____ avg. power _____

zone 1____ 2____ 3____ 4____ 5____

WORKOUT 2 S B R O _____

planned workout _____

_____

_____

route _____ dist. _____ time _____

avg. HR _____ avg. power _____

zone 1____ 2____ 3____ 4____ 5____

notes _____

_____

_____

_____

_____

_____

_____

_____

_____

nutrition _____

_____

_____

_____

120

SUNDAY _____ / ___ / _____

▦ sleep ▦ fatigue ▦ stress ▦ soreness

resting heart rate_____ weight _____

WORKOUT 1 S B R O _____

planned workout_____

_____

_____

route _____dist. _____time _____

avg. HR_____avg. power _____

zone 1_____ 2_____ 3_____ 4_____ 5_____

WORKOUT 2 S B R O _____

planned workout_____

_____

route _____dist. _____time _____

avg. HR_____avg. power _____

zone 1_____ 2_____ 3_____ 4_____ 5_____

notes _____

_____

_____

_____

_____

_____

_____

_____

_____

_____

_____

_____

nutrition _____

_____

_____

_____

WEEKLY SUMMARY

	time	distance	YTD time	YTD distance
swim				
bike				
run				
strength				
other				
total				

notes

_____

_____

_____

_____

_____

_____

_____

_____

period: _____   planned hours: _____

MONDAY _____ / _____ / _____

▢ sleep ▢ fatigue ▢ stress ▢ soreness

resting heart rate_____ weight _____

WORKOUT 1 S B R O _____

planned workout _____

_____

route _____ dist. _____ time _____

avg. HR _____ avg. power _____

zone 1_____ 2_____ 3_____ 4_____ 5_____

WORKOUT 2 S B R O _____

planned workout _____

_____

route _____ dist. _____ time _____

avg. HR _____ avg. power _____

zone 1_____ 2_____ 3_____ 4_____ 5_____

notes _____

_____

_____

_____

_____

_____

_____

_____

_____

_____

nutrition _____

_____

_____

_____

TUESDAY _____ / _____ / _____

▢ sleep ▢ fatigue ▢ stress ▢ soreness

resting heart rate_____ weight _____

WORKOUT 1 S B R O _____

planned workout _____

_____

route _____ dist. _____ time _____

avg. HR _____ avg. power _____

zone 1_____ 2_____ 3_____ 4_____ 5_____

WORKOUT 2 S B R O _____

planned workout _____

_____

route _____ dist. _____ time _____

avg. HR _____ avg. power _____

zone 1_____ 2_____ 3_____ 4_____ 5_____

notes _____

_____

_____

_____

_____

_____

_____

_____

_____

nutrition _____

_____

_____

_____

week goals: ▪ _____

▪ _____

▪ _____

WEDNESDAY ____ / ____ / ____

▪ sleep ▪ fatigue ▪ stress ▪ soreness

resting heart rate _____ weight _____

WORKOUT 1   S B R O _____

planned workout _____

_____

route _____ dist. _____ time _____

avg. HR _____ avg. power _____

zone 1 _____ 2 _____ 3 _____ 4 _____ 5 _____

WORKOUT 2   S B R O _____

planned workout _____

_____

route _____ dist. _____ time _____

avg. HR _____ avg. power _____

zone 1 _____ 2 _____ 3 _____ 4 _____ 5 _____

notes _____

_____

_____

_____

_____

_____

_____

_____

_____

_____

nutrition _____

_____

_____

_____

THURSDAY ____ / ____ / ____

▪ sleep ▪ fatigue ▪ stress ▪ soreness

resting heart rate _____ weight _____

WORKOUT 1   S B R O _____

planned workout _____

_____

route _____ dist. _____ time _____

avg. HR _____ avg. power _____

zone 1 _____ 2 _____ 3 _____ 4 _____ 5 _____

WORKOUT 2   S B R O _____

planned workout _____

_____

route _____ dist. _____ time _____

avg. HR _____ avg. power _____

zone 1 _____ 2 _____ 3 _____ 4 _____ 5 _____

notes _____

_____

_____

_____

_____

_____

_____

_____

nutrition _____

_____

_____

123

FRIDAY ___ / ___ / ___

▪ sleep ▪ fatigue ▪ stress ▪ soreness

resting heart rate_____ weight _____

WORKOUT 1 S B R O _____

planned workout _____

_____

_____

route _____ dist. _____ time _____

avg. HR _____ avg. power _____

zone 1_____ 2_____ 3_____ 4_____ 5_____

WORKOUT 2 S B R O _____

planned workout _____

_____

route _____ dist. _____ time _____

avg. HR _____ avg. power _____

zone 1_____ 2_____ 3_____ 4_____ 5_____

notes _____

_____

_____

_____

_____

_____

_____

_____

_____

_____

nutrition _____

_____

_____

SATURDAY ___ / ___ / ___

▪ sleep ▪ fatigue ▪ stress ▪ soreness

resting heart rate_____ weight _____

WORKOUT 1 S B R O _____

planned workout _____

_____

_____

route _____ dist. _____ time _____

avg. HR _____ avg. power _____

zone 1_____ 2_____ 3_____ 4_____ 5_____

WORKOUT 2 S B R O _____

planned workout _____

_____

route _____ dist. _____ time _____

avg. HR _____ avg. power _____

zone 1_____ 2_____ 3_____ 4_____ 5_____

notes _____

_____

_____

_____

_____

_____

_____

_____

_____

_____

nutrition _____

_____

_____

SUNDAY ___ / ___ / ___

☐ sleep ☐ fatigue ☐ stress ☐ soreness

resting heart rate _____ weight _____

WORKOUT 1 S B R O _____

planned workout _____

_____

_____

route _____ dist. _____ time _____

avg. HR _____ avg. power _____

zone 1 ____ 2 ____ 3 ____ 4 ____ 5 ____

WORKOUT 2 S B R O _____

planned workout _____

_____

route _____ dist. _____ time _____

avg. HR _____ avg. power _____

zone 1 ____ 2 ____ 3 ____ 4 ____ 5 ____

notes _____

_____

_____

_____

_____

_____

_____

_____

_____

_____

_____

_____

nutrition _____

_____

_____

WEEKLY SUMMARY

	time	distance	YTD time	YTD distance
swim				
bike				
run				
strength				
other				
total				

notes

_____

_____

_____

_____

_____

_____

_____

_____

period: _____   planned hours: _____

MONDAY _____ / _____ /

▓ sleep ▓ fatigue ▓ stress ▓ soreness

resting heart rate_____ weight _____

WORKOUT 1 S B R O _____

planned workout _____

_____

route _____ dist. _____ time _____

avg. HR _____ avg. power _____

zone 1_____ 2_____ 3_____ 4_____ 5_____

WORKOUT 2 S B R O _____

planned workout _____

_____

route _____ dist. _____ time _____

avg. HR _____ avg. power _____

zone 1_____ 2_____ 3_____ 4_____ 5_____

notes _____
_____
_____
_____
_____
_____
_____
_____
_____
_____
_____

nutrition _____
_____
_____
_____

TUESDAY _____ / _____ /

▓ sleep ▓ fatigue ▓ stress ▓ soreness

resting heart rate_____ weight _____

WORKOUT 1 S B R O _____

planned workout _____

_____

route _____ dist. _____ time _____

avg. HR _____ avg. power _____

zone 1_____ 2_____ 3_____ 4_____ 5_____

WORKOUT 2 S B R O _____

planned workout _____

_____

route _____ dist. _____ time _____

avg. HR _____ avg. power _____

zone 1_____ 2_____ 3_____ 4_____ 5_____

notes _____
_____
_____
_____
_____
_____
_____
_____
_____

nutrition _____
_____
_____

week goals: ▪ _____

▪ _____

▪ _____

WEDNESDAY _____ / _____ / _____

▪ sleep ▪ fatigue ▪ stress ▪ soreness

resting heart rate_____ weight _____

WORKOUT 1   S B R O _____

planned workout_____

_____

route _____ dist. _____ time _____

avg. HR_____ avg. power_____

zone 1_____ 2_____ 3_____ 4_____ 5_____

WORKOUT 2   S B R O _____

planned workout_____

_____

route _____ dist. _____ time _____

avg. HR_____ avg. power_____

zone 1_____ 2_____ 3_____ 4_____ 5_____

notes _____

_____

_____

_____

_____

_____

_____

_____

_____

_____

nutrition _____

_____

_____

THURSDAY _____ / _____ / _____

▪ sleep ▪ fatigue ▪ stress ▪ soreness

resting heart rate_____ weight _____

WORKOUT 1   S B R O _____

planned workout_____

_____

route _____ dist. _____ time _____

avg. HR_____ avg. power_____

zone 1_____ 2_____ 3_____ 4_____ 5_____

WORKOUT 2   S B R O _____

planned workout_____

_____

route _____ dist. _____ time _____

avg. HR_____ avg. power_____

zone 1_____ 2_____ 3_____ 4_____ 5_____

notes _____

_____

_____

_____

_____

_____

_____

_____

_____

_____

nutrition _____

_____

_____

FRIDAY ___/___/___

■ sleep ■ fatigue ■ stress ■ soreness

resting heart rate_____weight_____

WORKOUT 1 S B R O _____

planned workout_____

_____

_____

route _____dist._____time _____

avg. HR_____avg. power_____

zone 1_____2_____3_____4_____5_____

WORKOUT 2 S B R O _____

planned workout_____

_____

route _____dist._____time _____

avg. HR_____avg. power_____

zone 1_____2_____3_____4_____5_____

notes _____

_____

_____

_____

_____

_____

_____

_____

_____

_____

_____

_____

nutrition _____

_____

_____

_____

SATURDAY ___/___/___

■ sleep ■ fatigue ■ stress ■ soreness

resting heart rate_____weight_____

WORKOUT 1 S B R O _____

planned workout_____

_____

_____

route _____dist._____time _____

avg. HR_____avg. power_____

zone 1_____2_____3_____4_____5_____

WORKOUT 2 S B R O _____

planned workout_____

_____

route _____dist._____time _____

avg. HR_____avg. power_____

zone 1_____2_____3_____4_____5_____

notes _____

_____

_____

_____

_____

_____

_____

_____

_____

_____

_____

nutrition _____

_____

_____

SUNDAY ___ / ___ / ___

sleep ☐ fatigue ☐ stress ☐ soreness

resting heart rate _____ weight _____

WORKOUT 1 S B R O _____

planned workout _____

_____

_____

route _____ dist. _____ time _____

avg. HR _____ avg. power _____

zone 1____ 2____ 3____ 4____ 5____

WORKOUT 2 S B R O _____

planned workout _____

_____

route _____ dist. _____ time _____

avg. HR _____ avg. power _____

zone 1____ 2____ 3____ 4____ 5____

notes _____

_____

_____

_____

_____

_____

_____

_____

_____

_____

nutrition _____

_____

_____

_____

WEEKLY SUMMARY

	time	distance	YTD time	YTD distance
swim				
bike				
run				
strength				
other				
total				

notes

_____

_____

_____

_____

_____

_____

_____

_____

period: _____   planned hours: _____

MONDAY _____ / _____ / _____

☐ sleep ☐ fatigue ☐ stress ☐ soreness

resting heart rate _____ weight _____

WORKOUT 1 S B R O _____

planned workout _____

_____

route _____ dist. _____ time _____

avg. HR _____ avg. power _____

zone 1 ____ 2 ____ 3 ____ 4 ____ 5 ____

WORKOUT 2 S B R O _____

planned workout _____

_____

route _____ dist. _____ time _____

avg. HR _____ avg. power _____

zone 1 ____ 2 ____ 3 ____ 4 ____ 5 ____

notes _____

_____

_____

_____

_____

_____

_____

_____

_____

_____

nutrition _____

_____

_____

_____

TUESDAY _____ / _____ / _____

☐ sleep ☐ fatigue ☐ stress ☐ soreness

resting heart rate _____ weight _____

WORKOUT 1 S B R O _____

planned workout _____

_____

route _____ dist. _____ time _____

avg. HR _____ avg. power _____

zone 1 ____ 2 ____ 3 ____ 4 ____ 5 ____

WORKOUT 2 S B R O _____

planned workout _____

_____

route _____ dist. _____ time _____

avg. HR _____ avg. power _____

zone 1 ____ 2 ____ 3 ____ 4 ____ 5 ____

notes _____

_____

_____

_____

_____

_____

_____

_____

_____

_____

nutrition _____

_____

_____

_____

week goals: ▪ _____
▪ _____
▪ _____

WEDNESDAY _____ / _____ / _____

▪ sleep ▪ fatigue ▪ stress ▪ soreness

resting heart rate_____ weight _____

WORKOUT 1 S B R O _____

planned workout_____

_____

route _____ dist. _____ time _____

avg. HR_____ avg. power_____

zone 1_____ 2_____ 3_____ 4_____ 5_____

WORKOUT 2 S B R O _____

planned workout_____

_____

route _____ dist. _____ time _____

avg. HR_____ avg. power_____

zone 1_____ 2_____ 3_____ 4_____ 5_____

notes _____
_____
_____
_____
_____
_____
_____
_____
_____
_____

nutrition _____
_____
_____
_____

THURSDAY _____ / _____ / _____

▪ sleep ▪ fatigue ▪ stress ▪ soreness

resting heart rate_____ weight _____

WORKOUT 1 S B R O _____

planned workout_____

_____

route _____ dist. _____ time _____

avg. HR_____ avg. power_____

zone 1_____ 2_____ 3_____ 4_____ 5_____

WORKOUT 2 S B R O _____

planned workout_____

_____

route _____ dist. _____ time _____

avg. HR_____ avg. power_____

zone 1_____ 2_____ 3_____ 4_____ 5_____

notes _____
_____
_____
_____
_____
_____
_____
_____
_____

nutrition _____
_____
_____
_____

FRIDAY ___ / ___ / ___

▢ sleep ▢ fatigue ▢ stress ▢ soreness

resting heart rate _____ weight _____

WORKOUT 1 S B R O _____

planned workout _____

_____

_____

route _____ dist. _____ time _____

avg. HR _____ avg. power _____

zone 1 ___ 2 ___ 3 ___ 4 ___ 5 ___

WORKOUT 2 S B R O _____

planned workout _____

_____

route _____ dist. _____ time _____

avg. HR _____ avg. power _____

zone 1 ___ 2 ___ 3 ___ 4 ___ 5 ___

notes _____

_____

_____

_____

_____

_____

_____

_____

_____

_____

nutrition _____

_____

_____

_____

SATURDAY ___ / ___ / ___

▢ sleep ▢ fatigue ▢ stress ▢ soreness

resting heart rate _____ weight _____

WORKOUT 1 S B R O _____

planned workout _____

_____

_____

route _____ dist. _____ time _____

avg. HR _____ avg. power _____

zone 1 ___ 2 ___ 3 ___ 4 ___ 5 ___

WORKOUT 2 S B R O _____

planned workout _____

_____

route _____ dist. _____ time _____

avg. HR _____ avg. power _____

zone 1 ___ 2 ___ 3 ___ 4 ___ 5 ___

notes _____

_____

_____

_____

_____

_____

_____

_____

_____

_____

nutrition _____

_____

_____

SUNDAY ____ / ____ / ____

▢ sleep ▢ fatigue ▢ stress ▢ soreness

resting heart rate _____ weight _____

WORKOUT 1 S B R O _____

planned workout _____

_____

_____

route _____ dist. _____ time _____

avg. HR _____ avg. power _____

zone 1 ____ 2 ____ 3 ____ 4 ____ 5 ____

WORKOUT 2 S B R O _____

planned workout _____

_____

route _____ dist. _____ time _____

avg. HR _____ avg. power _____

zone 1 ____ 2 ____ 3 ____ 4 ____ 5 ____

notes _____

_____

_____

_____

_____

_____

_____

_____

_____

_____

nutrition _____

_____

_____

_____

WEEKLY SUMMARY

	time	distance	YTD time	YTD distance
swim				
bike				
run				
strength				
other				
total				

notes

_____

_____

_____

_____

_____

_____

_____

_____

week beginning:

period: _____   planned hours: _____

MONDAY _____ / _____ / _____

□ sleep □ fatigue □ stress □ soreness

resting heart rate _____ weight _____

WORKOUT 1 S B R O _____

planned workout _____

_____

route _____ dist. _____ time _____

avg. HR _____ avg. power _____

zone 1 _____ 2 _____ 3 _____ 4 _____ 5 _____

WORKOUT 2 S B R O _____

planned workout _____

_____

route _____ dist. _____ time _____

avg. HR _____ avg. power _____

zone 1 _____ 2 _____ 3 _____ 4 _____ 5 _____

notes _____

_____

_____

_____

_____

_____

_____

_____

_____

_____

_____

_____

nutrition _____

_____

_____

_____

_____

TUESDAY _____ / _____ / _____

□ sleep □ fatigue □ stress □ soreness

resting heart rate _____ weight _____

WORKOUT 1 S B R O _____

planned workout _____

_____

route _____ dist. _____ time _____

avg. HR _____ avg. power _____

zone 1 _____ 2 _____ 3 _____ 4 _____ 5 _____

WORKOUT 2 S B R O _____

planned workout _____

_____

route _____ dist. _____ time _____

avg. HR _____ avg. power _____

zone 1 _____ 2 _____ 3 _____ 4 _____ 5 _____

notes _____

_____

_____

_____

_____

_____

_____

_____

_____

_____

_____

nutrition _____

_____

_____

_____

week goals: ▪ _____

▪ _____

▪ _____

WEDNESDAY _____ / _____ / _____

▪ sleep ▪ fatigue ▪ stress ▪ soreness

resting heart rate_____ weight _____

WORKOUT 1 S B R O _____

planned workout _____

_____

route _____ dist. _____ time _____

avg. HR _____ avg. power _____

zone 1_____ 2_____ 3_____ 4_____ 5_____

WORKOUT 2 S B R O _____

planned workout _____

_____

route _____ dist. _____ time _____

avg. HR _____ avg. power _____

zone 1_____ 2_____ 3_____ 4_____ 5_____

notes _____

_____

_____

_____

_____

_____

_____

_____

_____

_____

nutrition _____

_____

_____

THURSDAY _____ / _____ / _____

▪ sleep ▪ fatigue ▪ stress ▪ soreness

resting heart rate_____ weight _____

WORKOUT 1 S B R O _____

planned workout _____

_____

route _____ dist. _____ time _____

avg. HR _____ avg. power _____

zone 1_____ 2_____ 3_____ 4_____ 5_____

WORKOUT 2 S B R O _____

planned workout _____

_____

route _____ dist. _____ time _____

avg. HR _____ avg. power _____

zone 1_____ 2_____ 3_____ 4_____ 5_____

notes _____

_____

_____

_____

_____

_____

_____

_____

_____

_____

nutrition _____

_____

_____

FRIDAY _____ / / _____

☐ sleep ☐ fatigue ☐ stress ☐ soreness

resting heart rate _____ weight _____

WORKOUT 1 S B R O _____

planned workout _____

_____

_____

route _____ dist. _____ time _____

avg. HR _____ avg. power _____

zone 1 _____ 2 _____ 3 _____ 4 _____ 5 _____

WORKOUT 2 S B R O _____

planned workout _____

_____

route _____ dist. _____ time _____

avg. HR _____ avg. power _____

zone 1 _____ 2 _____ 3 _____ 4 _____ 5 _____

notes _____

_____

_____

_____

_____

_____

_____

_____

_____

nutrition _____

_____

_____

_____

SATURDAY _____ / / _____

☐ sleep ☐ fatigue ☐ stress ☐ soreness

resting heart rate _____ weight _____

WORKOUT 1 S B R O _____

planned workout _____

_____

_____

route _____ dist. _____ time _____

avg. HR _____ avg. power _____

zone 1 _____ 2 _____ 3 _____ 4 _____ 5 _____

WORKOUT 2 S B R O _____

planned workout _____

_____

route _____ dist. _____ time _____

avg. HR _____ avg. power _____

zone 1 _____ 2 _____ 3 _____ 4 _____ 5 _____

notes _____

_____

_____

_____

_____

_____

_____

_____

_____

nutrition _____

_____

_____

_____

SUNDAY ___ / ___ / ___

☐ sleep ☐ fatigue ☐ stress ☐ soreness

resting heart rate_____ weight _____

WORKOUT 1 S B R O _____

planned workout _____

_____

_____

route _____ dist. _____ time _____

avg. HR _____ avg. power _____

zone 1____ 2____ 3____ 4____ 5____

WORKOUT 2 S B R O _____

planned workout _____

_____

route _____ dist. _____ time _____

avg. HR _____ avg. power _____

zone 1____ 2____ 3____ 4____ 5____

notes _____

_____

_____

_____

_____

_____

_____

_____

_____

_____

_____

_____

nutrition _____

_____

_____

_____

WEEKLY SUMMARY

	time	distance	YTD time	YTD distance
swim				
bike				
run				
strength				
other				
total				

notes

_____

_____

_____

_____

_____

_____

_____

_____

_____

_____

period: _____   planned hours: _____

MONDAY _____ / _____ /_____

▨ sleep ▨ fatigue ▨ stress ▨ soreness

resting heart rate_____ weight _____

WORKOUT 1 S B R O _____

planned workout _____

_____

route _____ dist. _____ time _____

avg. HR_____ avg. power _____

zone 1_____ 2_____ 3_____ 4_____ 5_____

WORKOUT 2 S B R O _____

planned workout _____

_____

route _____ dist. _____ time _____

avg. HR_____ avg. power _____

zone 1_____ 2_____ 3_____ 4_____ 5_____

notes _____

_____

_____

_____

_____

_____

_____

_____

_____

_____

nutrition _____

_____

_____

_____

TUESDAY _____ / _____ /_____

▨ sleep ▨ fatigue ▨ stress ▨ soreness

resting heart rate_____ weight _____

WORKOUT 1 S B R O _____

planned workout _____

_____

route _____ dist. _____ time _____

avg. HR_____ avg. power _____

zone 1_____ 2_____ 3_____ 4_____ 5_____

WORKOUT 2 S B R O _____

planned workout _____

_____

route _____ dist. _____ time _____

avg. HR_____ avg. power _____

zone 1_____ 2_____ 3_____ 4_____ 5_____

notes _____

_____

_____

_____

_____

_____

_____

_____

_____

nutrition _____

_____

_____

_____

week goals: ▪ _____

▪ _____

▪ _____

WEDNESDAY ____ / ____ / ____

▪ sleep ▪ fatigue ▪ stress ▪ soreness

resting heart rate_____ weight _____

WORKOUT 1 S B R O _____

planned workout _____

_____

route _____dist._____time _____

avg. HR_____avg. power_____

zone 1_____ 2_____ 3_____ 4_____ 5_____

WORKOUT 2 S B R O _____

planned workout _____

_____

route _____dist._____time _____

avg. HR_____avg. power_____

zone 1_____ 2_____ 3_____ 4_____ 5_____

notes _____

_____

_____

_____

_____

_____

_____

_____

_____

_____

nutrition _____

_____

_____

_____

THURSDAY ____ / ____ / ____

▪ sleep ▪ fatigue ▪ stress ▪ soreness

resting heart rate_____ weight _____

WORKOUT 1 S B R O _____

planned workout _____

_____

route _____dist._____time _____

avg. HR_____avg. power_____

zone 1_____ 2_____ 3_____ 4_____ 5_____

WORKOUT 2 S B R O _____

planned workout _____

_____

route _____dist._____time _____

avg. HR_____avg. power_____

zone 1_____ 2_____ 3_____ 4_____ 5_____

notes _____

_____

_____

_____

_____

_____

_____

_____

_____

_____

nutrition _____

_____

_____

FRIDAY _____ / ___ / _____

■ sleep ■ fatigue ■ stress ■ soreness

resting heart rate_____ weight _____

WORKOUT 1 S B R O _____

planned workout _____

_____

_____

route _____ dist. _____ time _____

avg. HR_____ avg. power _____

zone 1_____ 2_____ 3_____ 4_____ 5_____

WORKOUT 2 S B R O _____

planned workout _____

_____

route _____ dist. _____ time _____

avg. HR_____ avg. power _____

zone 1_____ 2_____ 3_____ 4_____ 5_____

notes _____

_____

_____

_____

_____

_____

_____

_____

_____

_____

nutrition _____

_____

_____

_____

SATURDAY _____ / ___ / _____

■ sleep ■ fatigue ■ stress ■ soreness

resting heart rate_____ weight _____

WORKOUT 1 S B R O _____

planned workout _____

_____

_____

route _____ dist. _____ time _____

avg. HR_____ avg. power _____

zone 1_____ 2_____ 3_____ 4_____ 5_____

WORKOUT 2 S B R O _____

planned workout _____

_____

_____

route _____ dist. _____ time _____

avg. HR_____ avg. power _____

zone 1_____ 2_____ 3_____ 4_____ 5_____

notes _____

_____

_____

_____

_____

_____

_____

_____

_____

_____

nutrition _____

_____

_____

SUNDAY _____ / ___ / _____

☐ sleep ☐ fatigue ☐ stress ☐ soreness

resting heart rate_____ weight _____

WORKOUT 1 S B R O _____

planned workout _____

_____

_____

route _____ dist. _____ time _____

avg. HR _____ avg. power _____

zone 1 ____ 2 ____ 3 ____ 4 ____ 5 ____

WORKOUT 2 S B R O _____

planned workout _____

_____

route _____ dist. _____ time _____

avg. HR _____ avg. power _____

zone 1 ____ 2 ____ 3 ____ 4 ____ 5 ____

notes _____

_____

_____

_____

_____

_____

_____

_____

_____

nutrition _____

_____

_____

_____

WEEKLY SUMMARY

	time	distance	YTD time	YTD distance
swim				
bike				
run				
strength				
other				
total				

notes

_____

_____

_____

_____

_____

_____

_____

_____

period: _____   planned hours: _____

MONDAY _____ / _____ /   notes _____

☐ sleep ☐ fatigue ☐ stress ☐ soreness   _____

resting heart rate_____ weight _____   _____

WORKOUT 1 S B R O _____   _____

planned workout _____   _____

_____   _____

route _____ dist. _____ time _____   _____

avg. HR _____ avg. power _____   _____

zone 1____ 2____ 3____ 4____ 5____   _____

WORKOUT 2 S B R O _____   _____

planned workout _____   _____

_____   **nutrition** _____

route _____ dist. _____ time _____   _____

avg. HR _____ avg. power _____   _____

zone 1____ 2____ 3____ 4____ 5____   _____

TUESDAY _____ / _____ /   notes _____

☐ sleep ☐ fatigue ☐ stress ☐ soreness   _____

resting heart rate_____ weight _____   _____

WORKOUT 1 S B R O _____   _____

planned workout _____   _____

_____   _____

route _____ dist. _____ time _____   _____

avg. HR _____ avg. power _____   _____

zone 1____ 2____ 3____ 4____ 5____   _____

WORKOUT 2 S B R O _____   _____

planned workout _____   _____

_____   **nutrition** _____

route _____ dist. _____ time _____   _____

avg. HR _____ avg. power _____   _____

zone 1____ 2____ 3____ 4____ 5____   _____

week goals: ▪ _____
▪ _____
▪ _____

WEDNESDAY ____ / ____ / ____   **notes** _____

▪ sleep ▪ fatigue ▪ stress ▪ soreness   _____

resting heart rate_____ weight _____   _____

WORKOUT 1 S B R O _____   _____

planned workout _____   _____

_____   _____

route _____ dist. _____ time _____   _____

avg. HR _____ avg. power _____   _____

zone 1____ 2____ 3____ 4____ 5____   _____

WORKOUT 2 S B R O _____   _____

planned workout _____   _____

_____   **nutrition** _____

route _____ dist. _____ time _____   _____

avg. HR _____ avg. power _____   _____

zone 1____ 2____ 3____ 4____ 5____   _____

THURSDAY ____ / ____ / ____   **notes** _____

▪ sleep ▪ fatigue ▪ stress ▪ soreness   _____

resting heart rate_____ weight _____   _____

WORKOUT 1 S B R O _____   _____

planned workout _____   _____

_____   _____

route _____ dist. _____ time _____   _____

avg. HR _____ avg. power _____   _____

zone 1____ 2____ 3____ 4____ 5____   _____

WORKOUT 2 S B R O _____   _____

planned workout _____   **nutrition** _____

_____   _____

route _____ dist. _____ time _____   _____

avg. HR _____ avg. power _____   _____

zone 1____ 2____ 3____ 4____ 5____   _____

FRIDAY ____ / ____ / _____

☐ sleep ☐ fatigue ☐ stress ☐ soreness

resting heart rate_____weight _____

WORKOUT 1   S B R O _____

planned workout_____

_____

_____

route _____dist. _____time _____

avg. HR_____avg. power _____

zone 1_____2_____ 3_____ 4_____ 5_____

WORKOUT 2 S B R O _____

planned workout_____

_____

route _____dist. _____time _____

avg. HR_____avg. power _____

zone 1_____2_____ 3_____ 4_____ 5_____

notes _____

_____

_____

_____

_____

_____

_____

_____

_____

_____

_____

nutrition _____

_____

_____

_____

SATURDAY ____ / ____ / _____

☐ sleep ☐ fatigue ☐ stress ☐ soreness

resting heart rate_____weight _____

WORKOUT 1   S B R O _____

planned workout_____

_____

_____

route _____dist. _____time _____

avg. HR_____avg. power _____

zone 1_____2_____ 3_____ 4_____ 5_____

WORKOUT 2 S B R O _____

planned workout_____

_____

_____

route _____dist. _____time _____

avg. HR_____avg. power _____

zone 1_____2_____ 3_____ 4_____ 5_____

notes _____

_____

_____

_____

_____

_____

_____

_____

_____

_____

_____

nutrition _____

_____

_____

SUNDAY _____ / ____ / ____

◻ sleep ◻ fatigue ◻ stress ◻ soreness

resting heart rate_____weight _____

WORKOUT 1 S B R O _____

planned workout_____

_____

_____

route _____dist. _____time _____

avg. HR_____avg. power_____

zone 1_____ 2_____ 3_____ 4_____ 5_____

WORKOUT 2 S B R O _____

planned workout_____

_____

route _____dist. _____time _____

avg. HR_____avg. power_____

zone 1_____ 2_____ 3_____ 4_____ 5_____

notes _____

_____

_____

_____

_____

_____

_____

_____

_____

_____

_____

nutrition _____

_____

_____

_____

WEEKLY SUMMARY

	time	distance	YTD time	YTD distance
swim				
bike				
run				
strength				
other				
total				

notes

_____

_____

_____

_____

_____

_____

_____

_____

period: _____   planned hours: _____

MONDAY _____ / _____ / _____

▨ sleep ▨ fatigue ▨ stress ▨ soreness

resting heart rate_____ weight _____

WORKOUT 1 S B R O _____

planned workout _____

_____

route _____ dist. _____ time _____

avg. HR _____ avg. power _____

zone 1_____ 2_____ 3_____ 4_____ 5_____

WORKOUT 2 S B R O _____

planned workout _____

_____

route _____ dist. _____ time _____

avg. HR _____ avg. power _____

zone 1_____ 2_____ 3_____ 4_____ 5_____

notes _____

_____
_____
_____
_____
_____
_____
_____
_____
_____
_____

nutrition _____

_____
_____
_____

TUESDAY _____ / _____ / _____

▨ sleep ▨ fatigue ▨ stress ▨ soreness

resting heart rate_____ weight _____

WORKOUT 1 S B R O _____

planned workout _____

_____

route _____ dist. _____ time _____

avg. HR _____ avg. power _____

zone 1_____ 2_____ 3_____ 4_____ 5_____

WORKOUT 2 S B R O _____

planned workout _____

_____

route _____ dist. _____ time _____

avg. HR _____ avg. power _____

zone 1_____ 2_____ 3_____ 4_____ 5_____

notes _____

_____
_____
_____
_____
_____
_____
_____
_____
_____

nutrition _____

_____
_____
_____

week goals: ▪ _____

▪ _____

▪ _____

WEDNESDAY ___ / ___ / ___

▪ sleep ▪ fatigue ▪ stress ▪ soreness

resting heart rate _____ weight _____

WORKOUT 1 S B R O _____

planned workout _____

_____

route _____ dist. _____ time _____

avg. HR _____ avg. power _____

zone 1____ 2____ 3____ 4____ 5____

WORKOUT 2 S B R O _____

planned workout _____

_____

route _____ dist. _____ time _____

avg. HR _____ avg. power _____

zone 1____ 2____ 3____ 4____ 5____

notes _____

_____

_____

_____

_____

_____

_____

_____

_____

_____

nutrition _____

_____

_____

_____

THURSDAY ___ / ___ / ___

▪ sleep ▪ fatigue ▪ stress ▪ soreness

resting heart rate _____ weight _____

WORKOUT 1 S B R O _____

planned workout _____

_____

route _____ dist. _____ time _____

avg. HR _____ avg. power _____

zone 1____ 2____ 3____ 4____ 5____

WORKOUT 2 S B R O _____

planned workout _____

_____

route _____ dist. _____ time _____

avg. HR _____ avg. power _____

zone 1____ 2____ 3____ 4____ 5____

notes _____

_____

_____

_____

_____

_____

_____

_____

_____

nutrition _____

_____

_____

_____

FRIDAY ___ / ___ / ___

■ sleep ■ fatigue ■ stress ■ soreness

resting heart rate_____ weight _____

WORKOUT 1 S B R O _____

planned workout _____

_____

_____

route _____ dist. _____ time _____

avg. HR _____ avg. power _____

zone 1____ 2____ 3____ 4____ 5____

WORKOUT 2 S B R O _____

planned workout _____

_____

route _____ dist. _____ time _____

avg. HR _____ avg. power _____

zone 1____ 2____ 3____ 4____ 5____

notes _____

_____

_____

_____

_____

_____

_____

_____

_____

_____

nutrition _____

_____

_____

_____

SATURDAY ___ / ___ / ___

■ sleep ■ fatigue ■ stress ■ soreness

resting heart rate_____ weight _____

WORKOUT 1 S B R O _____

planned workout _____

_____

_____

route _____ dist. _____ time _____

avg. HR _____ avg. power _____

zone 1____ 2____ 3____ 4____ 5____

WORKOUT 2 S B R O _____

planned workout _____

_____

route _____ dist. _____ time _____

avg. HR _____ avg. power _____

zone 1____ 2____ 3____ 4____ 5____

notes _____

_____

_____

_____

_____

_____

_____

_____

_____

_____

nutrition _____

_____

_____

SUNDAY ____ / ____ / ____

■ sleep ■ fatigue ■ stress ■ soreness

resting heart rate _____ weight _____

WORKOUT 1 S B R O _____

planned workout _____

_____

_____

route _____ dist. _____ time _____

avg. HR _____ avg. power _____

zone 1 _____ 2 _____ 3 _____ 4 _____ 5 _____

WORKOUT 2 S B R O _____

planned workout _____

_____

route _____ dist. _____ time _____

avg. HR _____ avg. power _____

zone 1 _____ 2 _____ 3 _____ 4 _____ 5 _____

notes _____

_____

_____

_____

_____

_____

_____

_____

_____

_____

nutrition _____

_____

_____

_____

WEEKLY SUMMARY

	time	distance	YTD time	YTD distance
swim				
bike				
run				
strength				
other				
total				

notes

_____

_____

_____

_____

_____

_____

_____

_____

period: _____ planned hours: _____

MONDAY _____ / _____ / _____

▢ sleep ▢ fatigue ▢ stress ▢ soreness

resting heart rate_____ weight _____

WORKOUT 1 S B R O _____

planned workout _____

_____

route _____dist. _____time _____

avg. HR_____avg. power_____

zone 1____2____3____4____5____

WORKOUT 2 S B R O _____

planned workout _____

_____

route _____dist. _____time _____

avg. HR_____avg. power_____

zone 1____2____3____4____5____

notes _____

_____

_____

_____

_____

_____

_____

_____

_____

_____

nutrition _____

_____

_____

_____

TUESDAY _____ / _____ / _____

▢ sleep ▢ fatigue ▢ stress ▢ soreness

resting heart rate_____ weight _____

WORKOUT 1 S B R O _____

planned workout _____

_____

route _____dist. _____time _____

avg. HR_____avg. power_____

zone 1____2____3____4____5____

WORKOUT 2 S B R O _____

planned workout _____

_____

route _____dist. _____time _____

avg. HR_____avg. power_____

zone 1____2____3____4____5____

notes _____

_____

_____

_____

_____

_____

_____

_____

_____

nutrition _____

_____

_____

_____

week goals: ▪ _____

▪ _____

▪ _____

WEDNESDAY ____ / ____ / ____

▪ sleep ▪ fatigue ▪ stress ▪ soreness

resting heart rate_____ weight _____

WORKOUT 1 S B R O _____

planned workout_____

_____

route _____dist. _____time _____

avg. HR_____avg. power_____

zone 1____ 2____ 3____ 4____ 5____

WORKOUT 2 S B R O _____

planned workout_____

_____

route _____dist. _____time _____

avg. HR_____avg. power_____

zone 1____ 2____ 3____ 4____ 5____

notes _____

_____

_____

_____

_____

_____

_____

_____

_____

_____

nutrition _____

_____

_____

_____

THURSDAY ____ / ____ / ____

▪ sleep ▪ fatigue ▪ stress ▪ soreness

resting heart rate_____ weight _____

WORKOUT 1 S B R O _____

planned workout_____

_____

route _____dist. _____time _____

avg. HR_____avg. power_____

zone 1____ 2____ 3____ 4____ 5____

WORKOUT 2 S B R O _____

planned workout_____

_____

route _____dist. _____time _____

avg. HR_____avg. power_____

zone 1____ 2____ 3____ 4____ 5____

notes _____

_____

_____

_____

_____

_____

_____

_____

_____

_____

nutrition _____

_____

_____

FRIDAY ___/___/___

▢ sleep ▢ fatigue ▢ stress ▢ soreness

resting heart rate_____ weight _____

WORKOUT 1   S B R O _____

planned workout _____

_____

_____

route _____ dist. _____ time _____

avg. HR _____ avg. power _____

zone 1____ 2____ 3____ 4____ 5____

WORKOUT 2 S B R O _____

planned workout _____

_____

route _____ dist. _____ time _____

avg. HR _____ avg. power _____

zone 1____ 2____ 3____ 4____ 5____

notes _____

_____

_____

_____

_____

_____

_____

_____

_____

_____

nutrition _____

_____

_____

_____

SATURDAY ___/___/___

▢ sleep ▢ fatigue ▢ stress ▢ soreness

resting heart rate_____ weight _____

WORKOUT 1   S B R O _____

planned workout _____

_____

_____

route _____ dist. _____ time _____

avg. HR _____ avg. power _____

zone 1____ 2____ 3____ 4____ 5____

WORKOUT 2 S B R O _____

planned workout _____

_____

route _____ dist. _____ time _____

avg. HR _____ avg. power _____

zone 1____ 2____ 3____ 4____ 5____

notes _____

_____

_____

_____

_____

_____

_____

_____

_____

_____

nutrition _____

_____

_____

SUNDAY ___ / ___ / ___

☐ sleep ☐ fatigue ☐ stress ☐ soreness

resting heart rate_____ weight _____

WORKOUT 1 S B R O _____

planned workout _____

_____

_____

route _____ dist. _____ time _____

avg. HR_____ avg. power _____

zone 1_____ 2 _____ 3 _____ 4 _____ 5 _____

WORKOUT 2 S B R O _____

planned workout _____

_____

route _____ dist. _____ time _____

avg. HR_____ avg. power _____

zone 1_____ 2 _____ 3 _____ 4 _____ 5 _____

notes _____

_____

_____

_____

_____

_____

_____

_____

_____

_____

_____

nutrition _____

_____

_____

WEEKLY SUMMARY

	time	distance	YTD time	YTD distance
swim				
bike				
run				
strength				
other				
total				

notes

_____

_____

_____

_____

_____

_____

_____

_____

period: _____   planned hours: _____

MONDAY _____ / ___ / _____   **notes** _____

☐ sleep ☐ fatigue ☐ stress ☐ soreness   _____

resting heart rate_____ weight _____   _____

WORKOUT 1 S B R O _____   _____

planned workout _____   _____

_____   _____

route _____ dist. _____ time _____   _____

avg. HR _____ avg. power _____   _____

zone 1_____ 2_____ 3_____ 4_____ 5_____   _____

WORKOUT 2 S B R O _____   _____

planned workout _____   _____

_____   **nutrition** _____

route _____ dist. _____ time _____   _____

avg. HR _____ avg. power _____   _____

zone 1_____ 2_____ 3_____ 4_____ 5_____   _____

TUESDAY _____ / ___ / _____   **notes** _____

☐ sleep ☐ fatigue ☐ stress ☐ soreness   _____

resting heart rate_____ weight _____   _____

WORKOUT 1 S B R O _____   _____

planned workout _____   _____

_____   _____

route _____ dist. _____ time _____   _____

avg. HR _____ avg. power _____   _____

zone 1_____ 2_____ 3_____ 4_____ 5_____   _____

WORKOUT 2 S B R O _____   _____

planned workout _____   _____

_____   **nutrition** _____

route _____ dist. _____ time _____   _____

avg. HR _____ avg. power _____   _____

zone 1_____ 2_____ 3_____ 4_____ 5_____   _____

week goals: ▪ _____

▪ _____

▪ _____

WEDNESDAY ____ / ____ / ____

▪ sleep ▪ fatigue ▪ stress ▪ soreness

resting heart rate_____ weight _____

WORKOUT 1 S B R O _____

planned workout _____

_____

route _____ dist. _____ time _____

avg. HR _____ avg. power _____

zone 1_____ 2_____ 3_____ 4_____ 5_____

WORKOUT 2 S B R O _____

planned workout _____

_____

route _____ dist. _____ time _____

avg. HR _____ avg. power _____

zone 1_____ 2_____ 3_____ 4_____ 5_____

notes _____

_____

_____

_____

_____

_____

_____

_____

_____

_____

nutrition _____

_____

_____

_____

THURSDAY ____ / ____ / ____

▪ sleep ▪ fatigue ▪ stress ▪ soreness

resting heart rate_____ weight _____

WORKOUT 1 S B R O _____

planned workout _____

_____

route _____ dist. _____ time _____

avg. HR _____ avg. power _____

zone 1_____ 2_____ 3_____ 4_____ 5_____

WORKOUT 2 S B R O _____

planned workout _____

_____

route _____ dist. _____ time _____

avg. HR _____ avg. power _____

zone 1_____ 2_____ 3_____ 4_____ 5_____

notes _____

_____

_____

_____

_____

_____

_____

_____

_____

nutrition _____

_____

_____

_____

FRIDAY ____ / ____ / ____

▩ sleep ▩ fatigue ▩ stress ▩ soreness

resting heart rate_____ weight _____

WORKOUT 1 S B R O _____

planned workout _____

_____

_____

route _____ dist. _____ time _____

avg. HR _____ avg. power _____

zone 1_____ 2_____ 3_____ 4_____ 5_____

WORKOUT 2 S B R O _____

planned workout _____

_____

route _____ dist. _____ time _____

avg. HR _____ avg. power _____

zone 1_____ 2_____ 3_____ 4_____ 5_____

notes _____

_____

_____

_____

_____

_____

_____

_____

_____

nutrition _____

_____

_____

SATURDAY ____ / ____ / ____

▩ sleep ▩ fatigue ▩ stress ▩ soreness

resting heart rate_____ weight _____

WORKOUT 1 S B R O _____

planned workout _____

_____

_____

route _____ dist. _____ time _____

avg. HR _____ avg. power _____

zone 1_____ 2_____ 3_____ 4_____ 5_____

WORKOUT 2 S B R O _____

planned workout _____

_____

_____

route _____ dist. _____ time _____

avg. HR _____ avg. power _____

zone 1_____ 2_____ 3_____ 4_____ 5_____

notes _____

_____

_____

_____

_____

_____

_____

_____

_____

_____

nutrition _____

_____

_____

SUNDAY _____ / ___ / ___

sleep ▓ fatigue ▓ stress ▓ soreness

resting heart rate_____ weight _____

WORKOUT 1 S B R O _____

planned workout_____

_____

_____

route _____ dist. _____ time _____

avg. HR_____ avg. power _____

zone 1____ 2____ 3____ 4____ 5____

WORKOUT 2 S B R O _____

planned workout_____

_____

route _____ dist. _____ time _____

avg. HR_____ avg. power _____

zone 1____ 2____ 3____ 4____ 5____

notes _____

_____

_____

_____

_____

_____

_____

_____

_____

_____

_____

nutrition _____

_____

_____

_____

WEEKLY SUMMARY

	time	distance	YTD time	YTD distance
swim				
bike				
run				
strength				
other				
total				

notes

_____

_____

_____

_____

_____

_____

_____

_____

week beginning: _____

period: _____   planned hours: _____

MONDAY _____ / _____ / _____

☐ sleep ☐ fatigue ☐ stress ☐ soreness

resting heart rate _____ weight _____

WORKOUT 1 S B R O _____

planned workout _____

_____

route _____ dist. _____ time _____

avg. HR _____ avg. power _____

zone 1 _____ 2 _____ 3 _____ 4 _____ 5 _____

WORKOUT 2 S B R O _____

planned workout _____

_____

route _____ dist. _____ time _____

avg. HR _____ avg. power _____

zone 1 _____ 2 _____ 3 _____ 4 _____ 5 _____

notes _____

_____

_____

_____

_____

_____

_____

_____

_____

nutrition _____

_____

_____

_____

TUESDAY _____ / _____ / _____

☐ sleep ☐ fatigue ☐ stress ☐ soreness

resting heart rate _____ weight _____

WORKOUT 1 S B R O _____

planned workout _____

_____

route _____ dist. _____ time _____

avg. HR _____ avg. power _____

zone 1 _____ 2 _____ 3 _____ 4 _____ 5 _____

WORKOUT 2 S B R O _____

planned workout _____

_____

route _____ dist. _____ time _____

avg. HR _____ avg. power _____

zone 1 _____ 2 _____ 3 _____ 4 _____ 5 _____

notes _____

_____

_____

_____

_____

_____

_____

_____

_____

nutrition _____

_____

_____

week goals: ▪ _____

▪ _____

▪ _____

WEDNESDAY _____ / _____ / _____

▪ sleep ▪ fatigue ▪ stress ▪ soreness

resting heart rate _____ weight _____

WORKOUT 1 S B R O _____

planned workout _____

_____

route _____ dist. _____ time _____

avg. HR _____ avg. power _____

zone 1_____ 2_____ 3_____ 4_____ 5_____

WORKOUT 2 S B R O _____

planned workout _____

_____

route _____ dist. _____ time _____

avg. HR _____ avg. power _____

zone 1_____ 2_____ 3_____ 4_____ 5_____

notes _____

_____

_____

_____

_____

_____

_____

_____

_____

_____

_____

nutrition _____

_____

_____

_____

THURSDAY _____ / _____ / _____

▪ sleep ▪ fatigue ▪ stress ▪ soreness

resting heart rate _____ weight _____

WORKOUT 1 S B R O _____

planned workout _____

_____

route _____ dist. _____ time _____

avg. HR _____ avg. power _____

zone 1_____ 2_____ 3_____ 4_____ 5_____

WORKOUT 2 S B R O _____

planned workout _____

_____

route _____ dist. _____ time _____

avg. HR _____ avg. power _____

zone 1_____ 2_____ 3_____ 4_____ 5_____

notes _____

_____

_____

_____

_____

_____

_____

_____

_____

_____

_____

nutrition _____

_____

_____

_____

FRIDAY _____ / ___ /

▨ sleep ▨ fatigue ▨ stress ▨ soreness

resting heart rate_____ weight _____

WORKOUT 1   S B R O _____

planned workout _____

_____

_____

route _____ dist. _____ time _____

avg. HR_____ avg. power_____

zone 1_____ 2_____ 3_____ 4_____ 5_____

WORKOUT 2   S B R O _____

planned workout _____

_____

nutrition _____

route _____ dist. _____ time _____

avg. HR_____ avg. power_____

zone 1_____ 2_____ 3_____ 4_____ 5_____

SATURDAY _____ / ___ /

notes _____

▨ sleep ▨ fatigue ▨ stress ▨ soreness

resting heart rate_____ weight _____

WORKOUT 1   S B R O _____

planned workout _____

_____

_____

route _____ dist. _____ time _____

avg. HR_____ avg. power_____

zone 1_____ 2_____ 3_____ 4_____ 5_____

WORKOUT 2   S B R O _____

planned workout _____

_____

nutrition _____

route _____ dist. _____ time _____

avg. HR_____ avg. power_____

zone 1_____ 2_____ 3_____ 4_____ 5_____

SUNDAY _____ / ____ / _____

☐ sleep ☐ fatigue ☐ stress ☐ soreness

resting heart rate _____ weight _____

WORKOUT 1 S B R O _____

planned workout _____

_____

_____

route _____ dist. _____ time _____

avg. HR _____ avg. power _____

zone 1 _____ 2 _____ 3 _____ 4 _____ 5 _____

WORKOUT 2 S B R O _____

planned workout _____

_____

route _____ dist. _____ time _____

avg. HR _____ avg. power _____

zone 1 _____ 2 _____ 3 _____ 4 _____ 5 _____

notes _____

_____

_____

_____

_____

_____

_____

_____

_____

_____

_____

_____

nutrition _____

_____

_____

_____

WEEKLY SUMMARY

	time	distance	YTD time	YTD distance
swim				
bike				
run				
strength				
other				
total				

notes

_____

_____

_____

_____

_____

_____

_____

_____

period: _____   planned hours: _____

MONDAY _____ / ____ / _____

◻ sleep ◻ fatigue ◻ stress ◻ soreness

resting heart rate_____ weight _____

WORKOUT 1 S B R O _____

planned workout _____

_____

route _____ dist. _____ time _____

avg. HR_____ avg. power_____

zone 1_____ 2_____ 3_____ 4_____ 5_____

WORKOUT 2 S B R O _____

planned workout _____

_____

route _____ dist. _____ time _____

avg. HR_____ avg. power_____

zone 1_____ 2_____ 3_____ 4_____ 5_____

notes _____

_____

_____

_____

_____

_____

_____

_____

_____

_____

nutrition _____

_____

_____

_____

TUESDAY _____ / ____ / _____

◻ sleep ◻ fatigue ◻ stress ◻ soreness

resting heart rate_____ weight _____

WORKOUT 1 S B R O _____

planned workout _____

_____

route _____ dist. _____ time _____

avg. HR_____ avg. power_____

zone 1_____ 2_____ 3_____ 4_____ 5_____

WORKOUT 2 S B R O _____

planned workout _____

_____

route _____ dist. _____ time _____

avg. HR_____ avg. power_____

zone 1_____ 2_____ 3_____ 4_____ 5_____

notes _____

_____

_____

_____

_____

_____

_____

_____

_____

_____

nutrition _____

_____

week goals: ▪ _____

▪ _____

▪ _____

WEDNESDAY ____ / ____ / ____

▪ sleep ▪ fatigue ▪ stress ▪ soreness

resting heart rate_____ weight _____

WORKOUT 1 S B R O _____

planned workout _____

_____

route _____ dist. _____ time _____

avg. HR _____ avg. power _____

zone 1____ 2____ 3____ 4____ 5____

WORKOUT 2 S B R O _____

planned workout _____

_____

route _____ dist. _____ time _____

avg. HR _____ avg. power _____

zone 1____ 2____ 3____ 4____ 5____

notes _____

_____

_____

_____

_____

_____

_____

_____

_____

_____

_____

nutrition _____

_____

_____

THURSDAY ____ / ____ / ____

▪ sleep ▪ fatigue ▪ stress ▪ soreness

resting heart rate_____ weight _____

WORKOUT 1 S B R O _____

planned workout _____

_____

route _____ dist. _____ time _____

avg. HR _____ avg. power _____

zone 1____ 2____ 3____ 4____ 5____

WORKOUT 2 S B R O _____

planned workout _____

_____

route _____ dist. _____ time _____

avg. HR _____ avg. power _____

zone 1____ 2____ 3____ 4____ 5____

notes _____

_____

_____

_____

_____

_____

_____

_____

_____

_____

nutrition _____

_____

_____

FRIDAY _____ / _____ / _____

☐ sleep ☐ fatigue ☐ stress ☐ soreness

resting heart rate _____ weight _____

WORKOUT 1 S B R O _____

planned workout _____

_____

_____

route _____ dist. _____ time _____

avg. HR _____ avg. power _____

zone 1 _____ 2 _____ 3 _____ 4 _____ 5 _____

WORKOUT 2 S B R O _____

planned workout _____

_____

_____

route _____ dist. _____ time _____

avg. HR _____ avg. power _____

zone 1 _____ 2 _____ 3 _____ 4 _____ 5 _____

notes _____

_____

_____

_____

_____

_____

_____

_____

_____

_____

nutrition _____

_____

_____

_____

SATURDAY _____ / _____ / _____

☐ sleep ☐ fatigue ☐ stress ☐ soreness

resting heart rate _____ weight _____

WORKOUT 1 S B R O _____

planned workout _____

_____

_____

route _____ dist. _____ time _____

avg. HR _____ avg. power _____

zone 1 _____ 2 _____ 3 _____ 4 _____ 5 _____

WORKOUT 2 S B R O _____

planned workout _____

_____

_____

route _____ dist. _____ time _____

avg. HR _____ avg. power _____

zone 1 _____ 2 _____ 3 _____ 4 _____ 5 _____

notes _____

_____

_____

_____

_____

_____

_____

_____

_____

_____

nutrition _____

_____

_____

SUNDAY _____ / _____ / _____

■ sleep ■ fatigue ■ stress ■ soreness

resting heart rate_____ weight _____

WORKOUT 1 S B R O _____

planned workout_____

_____

_____

route _____ dist. _____ time _____

avg. HR_____ avg. power_____

zone 1_____ 2_____ 3_____ 4_____ 5_____

WORKOUT 2 S B R O _____

planned workout_____

_____

route _____ dist. _____ time _____

avg. HR_____ avg. power_____

zone 1_____ 2_____ 3_____ 4_____ 5_____

notes _____

_____

_____

_____

_____

_____

_____

_____

_____

_____

_____

_____

nutrition _____

_____

_____

_____

WEEKLY SUMMARY

	time	distance	YTD time	YTD distance
swim				
bike				
run				
strength				
other				
total				

notes

_____

_____

_____

_____

_____

_____

_____

_____

_____

period: _____   planned hours: _____

MONDAY _____ / ____ / _____   notes _____

▢ sleep ▢ fatigue ▢ stress ▢ soreness   _____

resting heart rate_____ weight _____   _____

WORKOUT 1 S B R O _____   _____

planned workout_____   _____

_____   _____

route_____dist._____time _____   _____

avg. HR_____avg. power_____   _____

zone 1_____2_____3_____4_____5_____   _____

WORKOUT 2 S B R O _____   _____

planned workout_____   _____

_____   **nutrition** _____

route_____dist._____time _____   _____

avg. HR_____avg. power_____   _____

zone 1_____2_____3_____4_____5_____   _____

TUESDAY _____ / ____ / _____   notes _____

▢ sleep ▢ fatigue ▢ stress ▢ soreness   _____

resting heart rate_____ weight _____   _____

WORKOUT 1 S B R O _____   _____

planned workout_____   _____

_____   _____

route_____dist._____time _____   _____

avg. HR_____avg. power_____   _____

zone 1_____2_____3_____4_____5_____   _____

WORKOUT 2 S B R O _____   _____

planned workout_____   _____

_____   **nutrition** _____

route_____dist._____time _____   _____

avg. HR_____avg. power_____   _____

zone 1_____2_____3_____4_____5_____   _____

week goals: ▪ _____

▪ _____

▪ _____

WEDNESDAY ____ / ____ / ____

▪ sleep ▪ fatigue ▪ stress ▪ soreness

resting heart rate_____ weight _____

WORKOUT 1 S B R O _____

planned workout_____

_____

route _____dist._____time _____

avg. HR_____avg. power_____

zone 1_____ 2_____ 3_____ 4_____ 5_____

WORKOUT 2 S B R O _____

planned workout_____

_____

route _____dist._____time _____

avg. HR_____avg. power_____

zone 1_____ 2_____ 3_____ 4_____ 5_____

notes _____

_____

_____

_____

_____

_____

_____

_____

_____

nutrition _____

_____

_____

_____

THURSDAY ____ / ____ / ____

▪ sleep ▪ fatigue ▪ stress ▪ soreness

resting heart rate_____ weight _____

WORKOUT 1 S B R O _____

planned workout_____

_____

route _____dist._____time _____

avg. HR_____avg. power_____

zone 1_____ 2_____ 3_____ 4_____ 5_____

WORKOUT 2 S B R O _____

planned workout_____

_____

route _____dist._____time _____

avg. HR_____avg. power_____

zone 1_____ 2_____ 3_____ 4_____ 5_____

notes _____

_____

_____

_____

_____

_____

_____

_____

_____

nutrition _____

_____

_____

_____

FRIDAY ___ / ___ / ___

■ sleep ■ fatigue ■ stress ■ soreness

resting heart rate_____ weight _____

WORKOUT 1 S B R O _____

planned workout _____

_____

_____

route _____ dist. _____ time _____

avg. HR _____ avg. power _____

zone 1_____ 2_____ 3_____ 4_____ 5_____

WORKOUT 2 S B R O _____

planned workout _____

_____

route _____ dist. _____ time _____

avg. HR _____ avg. power _____

zone 1_____ 2_____ 3_____ 4_____ 5_____

notes _____

_____

_____

_____

_____

_____

_____

_____

_____

_____

nutrition _____

_____

_____

_____

SATURDAY ___ / ___ / ___

■ sleep ■ fatigue ■ stress ■ soreness

resting heart rate_____ weight _____

WORKOUT 1 S B R O _____

planned workout _____

_____

_____

route _____ dist. _____ time _____

avg. HR _____ avg. power _____

zone 1_____ 2_____ 3_____ 4_____ 5_____

WORKOUT 2 S B R O _____

planned workout _____

_____

_____

route _____ dist. _____ time _____

avg. HR _____ avg. power _____

zone 1_____ 2_____ 3_____ 4_____ 5_____

notes _____

_____

_____

_____

_____

_____

_____

_____

_____

_____

nutrition _____

_____

_____

_____

SUNDAY _____ / _____ / _____

☐ sleep ☐ fatigue ☐ stress ☐ soreness

resting heart rate_____ weight _____

WORKOUT 1 S B R O _____

planned workout_____

_____

_____

route _____dist. _____time _____

avg. HR_____avg. power_____

zone 1_____2_____3_____4_____5_____

WORKOUT 2 S B R O _____

planned workout_____

_____

route _____dist. _____time _____

avg. HR_____avg. power_____

zone 1_____2_____3_____4_____5_____

notes _____

_____

_____

_____

_____

_____

_____

_____

_____

_____

_____

_____

_____

nutrition _____

_____

_____

_____

WEEKLY SUMMARY

	time	distance	YTD time	YTD distance
swim				
bike				
run				
strength				
other				
total				

notes

_____

_____

_____

_____

_____

_____

_____

_____

_____

period: _____   planned hours: _____

MONDAY _____ / _____ / _____

■ sleep ■ fatigue ■ stress ■ soreness

resting heart rate_____ weight _____

WORKOUT 1 S B R O _____

planned workout_____

_____

route _____dist. _____time _____

avg. HR_____avg. power_____

zone 1_____ 2_____ 3_____ 4_____ 5_____

WORKOUT 2 S B R O _____

planned workout_____

_____

route _____dist. _____time _____

avg. HR_____avg. power_____

zone 1_____ 2_____ 3_____ 4_____ 5_____

notes _____

_____

_____

_____

_____

_____

_____

_____

_____

nutrition _____

_____

_____

_____

TUESDAY _____ / _____ / _____

■ sleep ■ fatigue ■ stress ■ soreness

resting heart rate_____ weight _____

WORKOUT 1 S B R O _____

planned workout_____

_____

route _____dist. _____time _____

avg. HR_____avg. power_____

zone 1_____ 2_____ 3_____ 4_____ 5_____

WORKOUT 2 S B R O _____

planned workout_____

_____

route _____dist. _____time _____

avg. HR_____avg. power_____

zone 1_____ 2_____ 3_____ 4_____ 5_____

notes _____

_____

_____

_____

_____

_____

_____

_____

_____

nutrition _____

_____

_____

_____

week goals: ▪ _____
▪ _____
▪ _____

WEDNESDAY ____ / ____ / ____

▪ sleep ▪ fatigue ▪ stress ▪ soreness

resting heart rate_____ weight _____

WORKOUT 1 S B R O _____

planned workout _____
_____

route _____ dist. _____ time _____
avg. HR _____ avg. power _____
zone 1____ 2 ____ 3 ____ 4____ 5____

WORKOUT 2 S B R O _____

planned workout _____
_____

route _____ dist. _____ time _____
avg. HR _____ avg. power _____
zone 1____ 2 ____ 3 ____ 4____ 5____

notes _____
_____
_____
_____
_____
_____
_____
_____
_____
_____

nutrition _____
_____
_____
_____

THURSDAY ____ / ____ / ____

▪ sleep ▪ fatigue ▪ stress ▪ soreness

resting heart rate_____ weight _____

WORKOUT 1 S B R O _____

planned workout _____
_____

route _____ dist. _____ time _____
avg. HR _____ avg. power _____
zone 1____ 2 ____ 3 ____ 4____ 5____

WORKOUT 2 S B R O _____

planned workout _____
_____

route _____ dist. _____ time _____
avg. HR _____ avg. power _____
zone 1____ 2 ____ 3 ____ 4____ 5____

notes _____
_____
_____
_____
_____
_____
_____
_____
_____

nutrition _____
_____
_____
_____

FRIDAY _____ / ___ / _____

notes _____

■ sleep ■ fatigue ■ stress ■ soreness

resting heart rate _____ weight _____

WORKOUT 1 S B R O _____

planned workout _____

_____

_____

route _____ dist. _____ time _____

avg. HR _____ avg. power _____

zone 1 _____ 2 _____ 3 _____ 4 _____ 5 _____

WORKOUT 2 S B R O _____

planned workout _____

_____

nutrition _____

route _____ dist. _____ time _____

avg. HR _____ avg. power _____

zone 1 _____ 2 _____ 3 _____ 4 _____ 5 _____

SATURDAY _____ / ___ / _____

notes _____

■ sleep ■ fatigue ■ stress ■ soreness

resting heart rate _____ weight _____

WORKOUT 1 S B R O _____

planned workout _____

_____

_____

route _____ dist. _____ time _____

avg. HR _____ avg. power _____

zone 1 _____ 2 _____ 3 _____ 4 _____ 5 _____

WORKOUT 2 S B R O _____

planned workout _____

_____

nutrition _____

route _____ dist. _____ time _____

avg. HR _____ avg. power _____

zone 1 _____ 2 _____ 3 _____ 4 _____ 5 _____

SUNDAY _____ / ___ / _____

☐ sleep ☐ fatigue ☐ stress ☐ soreness

resting heart rate_____ weight _____

WORKOUT 1 S B R O _____

planned workout_____

_____

_____

route _____dist. _____time _____

avg. HR_____avg. power_____

zone 1_____ 2_____ 3_____ 4_____ 5_____

WORKOUT 2 S B R O _____

planned workout_____

_____

route _____dist. _____time _____

avg. HR_____avg. power_____

zone 1_____ 2_____ 3_____ 4_____ 5_____

notes _____

_____

_____

_____

_____

_____

_____

_____

_____

_____

_____

nutrition _____

_____

_____

_____

WEEKLY SUMMARY

	time	distance	YTD time	YTD distance
swim				
bike				
run				
strength				
other				
total				

notes

_____

_____

_____

_____

_____

_____

_____

_____

period: _____ planned hours: _____

MONDAY _____ / _____ / _____

▨ sleep ▨ fatigue ▨ stress ▨ soreness

resting heart rate_____ weight _____

WORKOUT 1 S B R O _____

planned workout _____

_____

route _____ dist. _____ time _____

avg. HR _____ avg. power _____

zone 1____ 2____ 3____ 4____ 5____

WORKOUT 2 S B R O _____

planned workout _____

_____

route _____ dist. _____ time _____

avg. HR _____ avg. power _____

zone 1____ 2____ 3____ 4____ 5____

notes _____

_____

_____

_____

_____

_____

_____

_____

_____

_____

_____

_____

nutrition _____

_____

_____

_____

TUESDAY _____ / _____ / _____

▨ sleep ▨ fatigue ▨ stress ▨ soreness

resting heart rate_____ weight _____

WORKOUT 1 S B R O _____

planned workout _____

_____

route _____ dist. _____ time _____

avg. HR _____ avg. power _____

zone 1____ 2____ 3____ 4____ 5____

WORKOUT 2 S B R O _____

planned workout _____

_____

route _____ dist. _____ time _____

avg. HR _____ avg. power _____

zone 1____ 2____ 3____ 4____ 5____

notes _____

_____

_____

_____

_____

_____

_____

_____

_____

_____

_____

nutrition _____

_____

week goals: ▪ _____

▪ _____

▪ _____

WEDNESDAY ____/____/____

▪ sleep ▪ fatigue ▪ stress ▪ soreness

resting heart rate _____ weight _____

WORKOUT 1 S B R O _____

planned workout _____

_____

route _____ dist. _____ time _____

avg. HR _____ avg. power _____

zone 1 _____ 2 _____ 3 _____ 4 _____ 5 _____

WORKOUT 2 S B R O _____

planned workout _____

_____

route _____ dist. _____ time _____

avg. HR _____ avg. power _____

zone 1 _____ 2 _____ 3 _____ 4 _____ 5 _____

notes _____

_____

_____

_____

_____

_____

_____

_____

_____

_____

_____

nutrition _____

_____

_____

_____

THURSDAY ____/____/____

▪ sleep ▪ fatigue ▪ stress ▪ soreness

resting heart rate _____ weight _____

WORKOUT 1 S B R O _____

planned workout _____

_____

route _____ dist. _____ time _____

avg. HR _____ avg. power _____

zone 1 _____ 2 _____ 3 _____ 4 _____ 5 _____

WORKOUT 2 S B R O _____

planned workout _____

_____

route _____ dist. _____ time _____

avg. HR _____ avg. power _____

zone 1 _____ 2 _____ 3 _____ 4 _____ 5 _____

notes _____

_____

_____

_____

_____

_____

_____

_____

_____

_____

nutrition _____

_____

_____

_____

FRIDAY _____ / ___ / ___

◻ sleep ◻ fatigue ◻ stress ◻ soreness

resting heart rate_____ weight _____

WORKOUT 1 S B R O _____

planned workout _____

_____

_____

route _____ dist. _____ time _____

avg. HR _____ avg. power _____

zone 1_____ 2_____ 3_____ 4_____ 5_____

WORKOUT 2 S B R O _____

planned workout _____

_____

route _____ dist. _____ time _____

avg. HR _____ avg. power _____

zone 1_____ 2_____ 3_____ 4_____ 5_____

notes _____

_____

_____

_____

_____

_____

_____

_____

_____

_____

_____

nutrition _____

_____

_____

_____

SATURDAY _____ / ___ / ___

◻ sleep ◻ fatigue ◻ stress ◻ soreness

resting heart rate_____ weight _____

WORKOUT 1 S B R O _____

planned workout _____

_____

_____

route _____ dist. _____ time _____

avg. HR _____ avg. power _____

zone 1_____ 2_____ 3_____ 4_____ 5_____

WORKOUT 2 S B R O _____

planned workout _____

_____

_____

route _____ dist. _____ time _____

avg. HR _____ avg. power _____

zone 1_____ 2_____ 3_____ 4_____ 5_____

notes _____

_____

_____

_____

_____

_____

_____

_____

_____

_____

_____

nutrition _____

_____

_____

_____

SUNDAY ____ / ____ / ____

sleep ▢ fatigue ▢ stress ▢ soreness ▢

resting heart rate _____ weight _____

WORKOUT 1 S B R O _____

planned workout _____

_____

_____

route _____ dist. _____ time _____

avg. HR _____ avg. power _____

zone 1 ____ 2 ____ 3 ____ 4 ____ 5 ____

WORKOUT 2 S B R O _____

planned workout _____

_____

route _____ dist. _____ time _____

avg. HR _____ avg. power _____

zone 1 ____ 2 ____ 3 ____ 4 ____ 5 ____

notes _____

_____

_____

_____

_____

_____

_____

_____

_____

_____

_____

nutrition _____

_____

_____

_____

WEEKLY SUMMARY

	time	distance	YTD time	YTD distance
swim				
bike				
run				
strength				
other				
total				

notes

_____

_____

_____

_____

_____

_____

_____

period: _____   planned hours: _____

MONDAY _____ / _____ / _____

▨ sleep ▨ fatigue ▨ stress ▨ soreness

resting heart rate_____ weight _____

WORKOUT 1 S B R O _____

planned workout_____

_____

route _____dist. _____time _____

avg. HR_____avg. power_____

zone 1_____2_____3_____4_____5_____

WORKOUT 2 S B R O _____

planned workout_____

_____

route _____dist. _____time _____

avg. HR_____avg. power_____

zone 1_____2_____3_____4_____5_____

notes _____
_____
_____
_____
_____
_____
_____
_____
_____
_____

nutrition _____
_____
_____
_____

TUESDAY _____ / _____ / _____

▨ sleep ▨ fatigue ▨ stress ▨ soreness

resting heart rate_____ weight _____

WORKOUT 1 S B R O _____

planned workout_____

_____

route _____dist. _____time _____

avg. HR_____avg. power_____

zone 1_____2_____3_____4_____5_____

WORKOUT 2 S B R O _____

planned workout_____

_____

route _____dist. _____time _____

avg. HR_____avg. power_____

zone 1_____2_____3_____4_____5_____

notes _____
_____
_____
_____
_____
_____
_____
_____

nutrition _____
_____
_____

week goals: ▪ _____
▪ _____
▪ _____

WEDNESDAY ____ / ____ / ____

▪ sleep ▪ fatigue ▪ stress ▪ soreness

resting heart rate_____ weight _____

WORKOUT 1 S B R O _____

planned workout_____

_____

route _____ dist. _____ time _____
avg. HR _____ avg. power _____
zone 1____ 2____ 3____ 4____ 5____

WORKOUT 2 S B R O _____

planned workout_____

_____

route _____ dist. _____ time _____
avg. HR _____ avg. power _____
zone 1____ 2____ 3____ 4____ 5____

notes _____
_____
_____
_____
_____
_____
_____
_____
_____
_____

nutrition _____
_____
_____
_____

THURSDAY ____ / ____ / ____

▪ sleep ▪ fatigue ▪ stress ▪ soreness

resting heart rate_____ weight _____

WORKOUT 1 S B R O _____

planned workout_____

_____

route _____ dist. _____ time _____
avg. HR _____ avg. power _____
zone 1____ 2____ 3____ 4____ 5____

WORKOUT 2 S B R O _____

planned workout_____

_____

route _____ dist. _____ time _____
avg. HR _____ avg. power _____
zone 1____ 2____ 3____ 4____ 5____

notes _____
_____
_____
_____
_____
_____
_____
_____
_____

nutrition _____
_____
_____

FRIDAY _____ / ___ /_____

■ sleep ■ fatigue ■ stress ■ soreness

resting heart rate_____ weight _____

WORKOUT 1 S B R O _____

planned workout _____

_____

_____

route _____ dist. _____ time _____

avg. HR _____ avg. power _____

zone 1_____ 2_____ 3_____ 4_____ 5_____

WORKOUT 2 S B R O _____

planned workout _____

_____

route _____ dist. _____ time _____

avg. HR _____ avg. power _____

zone 1_____ 2_____ 3_____ 4_____ 5_____

notes _____

_____

_____

_____

_____

_____

_____

_____

_____

_____

nutrition _____

_____

_____

_____

SATURDAY _____ / ___ /_____

■ sleep ■ fatigue ■ stress ■ soreness

resting heart rate_____ weight _____

WORKOUT 1 S B R O _____

planned workout _____

_____

_____

route _____ dist. _____ time _____

avg. HR _____ avg. power _____

zone 1_____ 2_____ 3_____ 4_____ 5_____

WORKOUT 2 S B R O _____

planned workout _____

_____

_____

route _____ dist. _____ time _____

avg. HR _____ avg. power _____

zone 1_____ 2_____ 3_____ 4_____ 5_____

notes _____

_____

_____

_____

_____

_____

_____

_____

_____

_____

nutrition _____

_____

_____

_____

SUNDAY _____ / _____ / _____

☐ sleep ☐ fatigue ☐ stress ☐ soreness

resting heart rate_____ weight _____

WORKOUT 1 S B R O _____

planned workout _____

_____

_____

route _____ dist. _____ time _____

avg. HR_____ avg. power _____

zone 1_____ 2_____ 3_____ 4_____ 5_____

WORKOUT 2 S B R O _____

planned workout _____

_____

route _____ dist. _____ time _____

avg. HR_____ avg. power _____

zone 1_____ 2_____ 3_____ 4_____ 5_____

notes _____

_____

_____

_____

_____

_____

_____

_____

_____

_____

_____

nutrition _____

_____

_____

_____

WEEKLY SUMMARY

	time	distance	YTD time	YTD distance
swim				
bike				
run				
strength				
other				
total				

notes

_____

_____

_____

_____

_____

_____

_____

_____

period: _____   planned hours: _____

MONDAY _____ / ___ / _____

☐ sleep ☐ fatigue ☐ stress ☐ soreness

resting heart rate_____ weight _____

WORKOUT 1 S B R O _____

planned workout _____

_____

route _____ dist. _____ time _____

avg. HR _____ avg. power _____

zone 1____ 2____ 3____ 4____ 5____

WORKOUT 2 S B R O _____

planned workout _____

_____

route _____ dist. _____ time _____

avg. HR _____ avg. power _____

zone 1____ 2____ 3____ 4____ 5____

notes _____

_____

_____

_____

_____

_____

_____

_____

_____

_____

nutrition _____

_____

_____

_____

TUESDAY _____ / ___ / _____

☐ sleep ☐ fatigue ☐ stress ☐ soreness

resting heart rate_____ weight _____

WORKOUT 1 S B R O _____

planned workout _____

_____

route _____ dist. _____ time _____

avg. HR _____ avg. power _____

zone 1____ 2____ 3____ 4____ 5____

WORKOUT 2 S B R O _____

planned workout _____

_____

route _____ dist. _____ time _____

avg. HR _____ avg. power _____

zone 1____ 2____ 3____ 4____ 5____

notes _____

_____

_____

_____

_____

_____

_____

_____

_____

nutrition _____

_____

week goals: ▪ _____

▪ _____

▪ _____

WEDNESDAY ____ / ____ / ____

▪ sleep ▪ fatigue ▪ stress ▪ soreness

resting heart rate_____ weight _____

WORKOUT 1   S B R O _____

planned workout _____

_____

route _____ dist. _____ time _____

avg. HR_____ avg. power_____

zone 1_____ 2_____ 3_____ 4_____ 5_____

WORKOUT 2   S B R O _____

planned workout _____

_____

route _____ dist. _____ time _____

avg. HR_____ avg. power_____

zone 1_____ 2_____ 3_____ 4_____ 5_____

notes _____

_____

_____

_____

_____

_____

_____

_____

_____

nutrition _____

_____

_____

_____

THURSDAY ____ / ____ / ____

▪ sleep ▪ fatigue ▪ stress ▪ soreness

resting heart rate_____ weight _____

WORKOUT 1   S B R O _____

planned workout _____

_____

route _____ dist. _____ time _____

avg. HR_____ avg. power_____

zone 1_____ 2_____ 3_____ 4_____ 5_____

WORKOUT 2   S B R O _____

planned workout _____

_____

route _____ dist. _____ time _____

avg. HR_____ avg. power_____

zone 1_____ 2_____ 3_____ 4_____ 5_____

notes _____

_____

_____

_____

_____

_____

_____

_____

_____

nutrition _____

_____

_____

_____

FRIDAY _____ / ___ / _____

▨ sleep ▨ fatigue ▨ stress ▨ soreness

resting heart rate_____ weight _____

WORKOUT 1 S B R O _____

planned workout _____

_____

_____

route _____ dist. _____ time _____

avg. HR _____ avg. power _____

zone 1_____ 2 _____ 3 _____ 4 _____ 5 _____

WORKOUT 2 S B R O _____

planned workout _____

_____

route _____ dist. _____ time _____

avg. HR _____ avg. power _____

zone 1_____ 2 _____ 3 _____ 4 _____ 5 _____

notes _____

_____

_____

_____

_____

_____

_____

_____

_____

_____

_____

_____

nutrition _____

_____

_____

_____

SATURDAY _____ / ___ / _____

▨ sleep ▨ fatigue ▨ stress ▨ soreness

resting heart rate_____ weight _____

WORKOUT 1 S B R O _____

planned workout _____

_____

_____

route _____ dist. _____ time _____

avg. HR _____ avg. power _____

zone 1_____ 2 _____ 3 _____ 4 _____ 5 _____

WORKOUT 2 S B R O _____

planned workout _____

_____

route _____ dist. _____ time _____

avg. HR _____ avg. power _____

zone 1_____ 2 _____ 3 _____ 4 _____ 5 _____

notes _____

_____

_____

_____

_____

_____

_____

_____

_____

_____

_____

_____

nutrition _____

_____

_____

_____

SUNDAY _____ / ___ / _____

▨ sleep ▨ fatigue ▨ stress ▨ soreness

resting heart rate_____ weight _____

WORKOUT 1 S B R O _____

planned workout_____

_____

_____

route _____dist. _____time _____

avg. HR_____avg. power_____

zone 1_____2_____3_____4_____5_____

WORKOUT 2 S B R O _____

planned workout_____

_____

route _____dist. _____time _____

avg. HR_____avg. power_____

zone 1_____2_____3_____4_____5_____

notes _____

_____

_____

_____

_____

_____

_____

_____

_____

_____

_____

nutrition _____

_____

_____

_____

WEEKLY SUMMARY

	time	distance	YTD time	YTD distance
swim				
bike				
run				
strength				
other				
total				

notes

_____

_____

_____

_____

_____

_____

_____

_____

_____

period: _____   planned hours: _____

MONDAY _____ / _____ /_____   **notes** _____

░ sleep ░ fatigue ░ stress ░ soreness   _____

resting heart rate_____ weight _____   _____

WORKOUT 1 S B R O _____   _____

planned workout_____   _____

_____   _____

route _____dist. _____time _____   _____

avg. HR_____avg. power_____   _____

zone 1_____2_____3_____4_____5_____   _____

WORKOUT 2 S B R O _____   _____

planned workout_____   _____

_____   **nutrition** _____

route _____dist. _____time _____   _____

avg. HR_____avg. power_____   _____

zone 1_____2_____3_____4_____5_____   _____

TUESDAY _____ / _____ /_____   **notes** _____

░ sleep ░ fatigue ░ stress ░ soreness   _____

resting heart rate_____ weight _____   _____

WORKOUT 1 S B R O _____   _____

planned workout_____   _____

_____   _____

route _____dist. _____time _____   _____

avg. HR_____avg. power_____   _____

zone 1_____2_____3_____4_____5_____   _____

WORKOUT 2 S B R O _____   _____

planned workout_____   _____

_____   **nutrition** _____

route _____dist. _____time _____   _____

avg. HR_____avg. power_____   _____

zone 1_____2_____3_____4_____5_____   _____

week goals: ▪ _____

▪ _____

▪ _____

WEDNESDAY ____ / ____ / ____

▪ sleep ▪ fatigue ▪ stress ▪ soreness

resting heart rate_____ weight _____

WORKOUT 1 S B R O _____

planned workout _____

_____

route _____ dist. _____ time _____

avg. HR _____ avg. power _____

zone 1_____ 2_____ 3_____ 4_____ 5_____

WORKOUT 2 S B R O _____

planned workout _____

_____

route _____ dist. _____ time _____

avg. HR _____ avg. power _____

zone 1_____ 2_____ 3_____ 4_____ 5_____

notes _____

_____

_____

_____

_____

_____

_____

_____

_____

_____

_____

nutrition _____

_____

_____

_____

THURSDAY ____ / ____ / ____

▪ sleep ▪ fatigue ▪ stress ▪ soreness

resting heart rate_____ weight _____

WORKOUT 1 S B R O _____

planned workout _____

_____

route _____ dist. _____ time _____

avg. HR _____ avg. power _____

zone 1_____ 2_____ 3_____ 4_____ 5_____

WORKOUT 2 S B R O _____

planned workout _____

_____

route _____ dist. _____ time _____

avg. HR _____ avg. power _____

zone 1_____ 2_____ 3_____ 4_____ 5_____

notes _____

_____

_____

_____

_____

_____

_____

_____

_____

_____

_____

nutrition _____

_____

_____

FRIDAY _____ / /

☐ sleep ☐ fatigue ☐ stress ☐ soreness

resting heart rate _____ weight _____

WORKOUT 1 S B R O _____

planned workout _____

_____

_____

route _____ dist. _____ time _____

avg. HR _____ avg. power _____

zone 1____ 2____ 3____ 4____ 5____

WORKOUT 2 S B R O _____

planned workout _____

_____

route _____ dist. _____ time _____

avg. HR _____ avg. power _____

zone 1____ 2____ 3____ 4____ 5____

notes _____

_____

_____

_____

_____

_____

_____

_____

_____

nutrition _____

_____

_____

_____

SATURDAY _____ / /

☐ sleep ☐ fatigue ☐ stress ☐ soreness

resting heart rate _____ weight _____

WORKOUT 1 S B R O _____

planned workout _____

_____

_____

route _____ dist. _____ time _____

avg. HR _____ avg. power _____

zone 1____ 2____ 3____ 4____ 5____

WORKOUT 2 S B R O _____

planned workout _____

_____

_____

route _____ dist. _____ time _____

avg. HR _____ avg. power _____

zone 1____ 2____ 3____ 4____ 5____

notes _____

_____

_____

_____

_____

_____

_____

_____

_____

nutrition _____

_____

_____

_____

SUNDAY _____ / _____ / _____

■ sleep ■ fatigue ■ stress ■ soreness

resting heart rate _____ weight _____

WORKOUT 1 S B R O _____

planned workout _____

_____

_____

route _____ dist. _____ time _____

avg. HR _____ avg. power _____

zone 1 _____ 2 _____ 3 _____ 4 _____ 5 _____

WORKOUT 2 S B R O _____

planned workout _____

_____

route _____ dist. _____ time _____

avg. HR _____ avg. power _____

zone 1 _____ 2 _____ 3 _____ 4 _____ 5 _____

notes _____

_____

_____

_____

_____

_____

_____

_____

_____

_____

_____

nutrition _____

_____

_____

WEEKLY SUMMARY

	time	distance	YTD time	YTD distance
swim				
bike				
run				
strength				
other				
total				

notes

_____

_____

_____

_____

_____

_____

_____

_____

period: _____   planned hours: _____

MONDAY _____ / ___ / _____

▢ sleep ▢ fatigue ▢ stress ▢ soreness

resting heart rate_____ weight _____

WORKOUT 1 S B R O _____

planned workout _____

_____

route _____ dist. _____ time _____

avg. HR _____ avg. power _____

zone 1_____ 2_____ 3_____ 4_____ 5_____

WORKOUT 2 S B R O _____

planned workout _____

_____

route _____ dist. _____ time _____

avg. HR _____ avg. power _____

zone 1_____ 2_____ 3_____ 4_____ 5_____

notes _____

_____

_____

_____

_____

_____

_____

_____

_____

_____

nutrition _____

_____

_____

_____

TUESDAY _____ / ___ / _____

▢ sleep ▢ fatigue ▢ stress ▢ soreness

resting heart rate_____ weight _____

WORKOUT 1 S B R O _____

planned workout _____

_____

route _____ dist. _____ time _____

avg. HR _____ avg. power _____

zone 1_____ 2_____ 3_____ 4_____ 5_____

WORKOUT 2 S B R O _____

planned workout _____

_____

route _____ dist. _____ time _____

avg. HR _____ avg. power _____

zone 1_____ 2_____ 3_____ 4_____ 5_____

notes _____

_____

_____

_____

_____

_____

_____

_____

_____

_____

nutrition _____

_____

_____

week goals: ▪ _____
▪ _____
▪ _____

WEDNESDAY ___ / ___ / ___

▪ sleep ▪ fatigue ▪ stress ▪ soreness

resting heart rate_____ weight _____

WORKOUT 1 S B R O _____

planned workout_____
_____

route _____ dist. _____ time _____

avg. HR_____ avg. power_____

zone 1____ 2____ 3____ 4____ 5____

WORKOUT 2 S B R O _____

planned workout_____
_____

route _____ dist. _____ time _____

avg. HR_____ avg. power_____

zone 1____ 2____ 3____ 4____ 5____

notes _____
_____
_____
_____
_____
_____
_____
_____
_____

nutrition _____
_____
_____
_____

THURSDAY ___ / ___ / ___

▪ sleep ▪ fatigue ▪ stress ▪ soreness

resting heart rate_____ weight _____

WORKOUT 1 S B R O _____

planned workout_____
_____

route _____ dist. _____ time _____

avg. HR_____ avg. power_____

zone 1____ 2____ 3____ 4____ 5____

WORKOUT 2 S B R O _____

planned workout_____
_____

route _____ dist. _____ time _____

avg. HR_____ avg. power_____

zone 1____ 2____ 3____ 4____ 5____

notes _____
_____
_____
_____
_____
_____
_____
_____

nutrition _____
_____
_____

FRIDAY ____ / ____ / ____

☐ sleep ☐ fatigue ☐ stress ☐ soreness

resting heart rate _____ weight _____

WORKOUT 1 S B R O _____

planned workout _____

_____

_____

route _____ dist. _____ time _____

avg. HR _____ avg. power _____

zone 1 ____ 2 ____ 3 ____ 4 ____ 5 ____

WORKOUT 2 S B R O _____

planned workout _____

_____

route _____ dist. _____ time _____

avg. HR _____ avg. power _____

zone 1 ____ 2 ____ 3 ____ 4 ____ 5 ____

notes _____

_____

_____

_____

_____

_____

_____

_____

_____

_____

nutrition _____

_____

_____

_____

SATURDAY ____ / ____ / ____

☐ sleep ☐ fatigue ☐ stress ☐ soreness

resting heart rate _____ weight _____

WORKOUT 1 S B R O _____

planned workout _____

_____

_____

route _____ dist. _____ time _____

avg. HR _____ avg. power _____

zone 1 ____ 2 ____ 3 ____ 4 ____ 5 ____

WORKOUT 2 S B R O _____

planned workout _____

_____

_____

route _____ dist. _____ time _____

avg. HR _____ avg. power _____

zone 1 ____ 2 ____ 3 ____ 4 ____ 5 ____

notes _____

_____

_____

_____

_____

_____

_____

_____

_____

_____

_____

nutrition _____

_____

_____

SUNDAY ___ / ___ / ___

■ sleep ■ fatigue ■ stress ■ soreness

resting heart rate_____ weight _____

WORKOUT 1 S B R O _____

planned workout _____

_____

_____

route _____ dist. _____ time _____

avg. HR_____ avg. power _____

zone 1_____ 2_____ 3_____ 4_____ 5_____

WORKOUT 2 S B R O _____

planned workout _____

_____

route _____ dist. _____ time _____

avg. HR_____ avg. power _____

zone 1_____ 2_____ 3_____ 4_____ 5_____

notes _____

_____

_____

_____

_____

_____

_____

_____

_____

_____

_____

nutrition _____

_____

_____

WEEKLY SUMMARY

	time	distance	YTD time	YTD distance
swim				
bike				
run				
strength				
other				
total				

notes

_____

_____

_____

_____

_____

_____

_____

period: _____   planned hours: _____

MONDAY _____ / ____ / _____   notes _____

▨ sleep ▨ fatigue ▨ stress ▨ soreness   _____

resting heart rate_____ weight _____   _____

WORKOUT 1 S B R O _____   _____

planned workout_____   _____

_____   _____

route _____ dist. _____ time _____   _____

avg. HR_____ avg. power _____   _____

zone 1_____ 2_____ 3_____ 4_____ 5_____   _____

WORKOUT 2 S B R O _____   _____

planned workout_____   _____

_____   **nutrition** _____

route _____ dist. _____ time _____   _____

avg. HR_____ avg. power _____   _____

zone 1_____ 2_____ 3_____ 4_____ 5_____   _____

TUESDAY _____ / ____ / _____   notes _____

▨ sleep ▨ fatigue ▨ stress ▨ soreness   _____

resting heart rate_____ weight _____   _____

WORKOUT 1 S B R O _____   _____

planned workout_____   _____

_____   _____

route _____ dist. _____ time _____   _____

avg. HR_____ avg. power _____   _____

zone 1_____ 2_____ 3_____ 4_____ 5_____   _____

WORKOUT 2 S B R O _____   _____

planned workout_____   _____

_____   **nutrition** _____

route _____ dist. _____ time _____   _____

avg. HR_____ avg. power _____   _____

zone 1_____ 2_____ 3_____ 4_____ 5_____   _____

week goals: ■ _____

■ _____

■ _____

WEDNESDAY ___ / ___ / ___

■ sleep ■ fatigue ■ stress ■ soreness

resting heart rate_____ weight _____

WORKOUT 1 S B R O _____

planned workout _____

_____

route _____ dist. _____ time _____

avg. HR _____ avg. power _____

zone 1_____ 2_____ 3_____ 4_____ 5_____

WORKOUT 2 S B R O _____

planned workout _____

_____

route _____ dist. _____ time _____

avg. HR _____ avg. power _____

zone 1_____ 2_____ 3_____ 4_____ 5_____

notes _____

_____

_____

_____

_____

_____

_____

_____

_____

nutrition _____

_____

_____

_____

THURSDAY ___ / ___ / ___

■ sleep ■ fatigue ■ stress ■ soreness

resting heart rate_____ weight _____

WORKOUT 1 S B R O _____

planned workout _____

_____

route _____ dist. _____ time _____

avg. HR _____ avg. power _____

zone 1_____ 2_____ 3_____ 4_____ 5_____

WORKOUT 2 S B R O _____

planned workout _____

_____

route _____ dist. _____ time _____

avg. HR _____ avg. power _____

zone 1_____ 2_____ 3_____ 4_____ 5_____

notes _____

_____

_____

_____

_____

_____

_____

_____

_____

nutrition _____

_____

_____

_____

FRIDAY ___ / ___ /

■ sleep ■ fatigue ■ stress ■ soreness

resting heart rate_____ weight _____

WORKOUT 1 S B R O _____

planned workout_____

_____

_____

route _____ dist. _____ time _____

avg. HR _____ avg. power _____

zone 1_____ 2_____ 3_____ 4_____ 5_____

WORKOUT 2 S B R O _____

planned workout_____

_____

route _____ dist. _____ time _____

avg. HR _____ avg. power _____

zone 1_____ 2_____ 3_____ 4_____ 5_____

notes _____

_____

_____

_____

_____

_____

_____

_____

_____

_____

nutrition _____

_____

_____

_____

SATURDAY ___ / ___ /

■ sleep ■ fatigue ■ stress ■ soreness

resting heart rate_____ weight _____

WORKOUT 1 S B R O _____

planned workout_____

_____

_____

route _____ dist. _____ time _____

avg. HR _____ avg. power _____

zone 1_____ 2_____ 3_____ 4_____ 5_____

WORKOUT 2 S B R O _____

planned workout_____

_____

_____

route _____ dist. _____ time _____

avg. HR _____ avg. power _____

zone 1_____ 2_____ 3_____ 4_____ 5_____

notes _____

_____

_____

_____

_____

_____

_____

_____

_____

_____

nutrition _____

_____

_____

_____

SUNDAY ___ / ___ / ___

sleep fatigue stress soreness

resting heart rate_____ weight _____

WORKOUT 1 S B R O _____

planned workout_____

_____

_____

route _____ dist. _____ time _____

avg. HR_____ avg. power_____

zone 1_____ 2_____ 3_____ 4_____ 5_____

WORKOUT 2 S B R O _____

planned workout_____

_____

route _____ dist. _____ time _____

avg. HR_____ avg. power_____

zone 1_____ 2_____ 3_____ 4_____ 5_____

notes _____

_____

_____

_____

_____

_____

_____

_____

_____

nutrition _____

_____

_____

_____

WEEKLY SUMMARY

	time	distance	YTD time	YTD distance
swim				
bike				
run				
strength				
other				
total				

notes

_____

_____

_____

_____

_____

_____

_____

period: _____   planned hours: _____

MONDAY _____ / _____ / _____

▓ sleep ▓ fatigue ▓ stress ▓ soreness

resting heart rate _____ weight _____

WORKOUT 1 S B R O _____

planned workout _____

_____

route _____ dist. _____ time _____

avg. HR _____ avg. power _____

zone 1 ____ 2 ____ 3 ____ 4 ____ 5 ____

WORKOUT 2 S B R O _____

planned workout _____

_____

route _____ dist. _____ time _____

avg. HR _____ avg. power _____

zone 1 ____ 2 ____ 3 ____ 4 ____ 5 ____

notes _____

_____

_____

_____

_____

_____

_____

_____

_____

_____

_____

nutrition _____

_____

_____

_____

TUESDAY _____ / _____ / _____

▓ sleep ▓ fatigue ▓ stress ▓ soreness

resting heart rate _____ weight _____

WORKOUT 1 S B R O _____

planned workout _____

_____

route _____ dist. _____ time _____

avg. HR _____ avg. power _____

zone 1 ____ 2 ____ 3 ____ 4 ____ 5 ____

WORKOUT 2 S B R O _____

planned workout _____

_____

route _____ dist. _____ time _____

avg. HR _____ avg. power _____

zone 1 ____ 2 ____ 3 ____ 4 ____ 5 ____

notes _____

_____

_____

_____

_____

_____

_____

_____

_____

_____

_____

nutrition _____

_____

_____

week goals: ▪ _____

▪ _____

▪ _____

WEDNESDAY ____ / ____ / ____

▪ sleep ▪ fatigue ▪ stress ▪ soreness

resting heart rate_____ weight _____

WORKOUT 1 S B R O _____

planned workout_____

_____

route _____dist. _____time _____

avg. HR_____avg. power _____

zone 1_____2_____3_____4_____5_____

WORKOUT 2 S B R O _____

planned workout_____

_____

route _____dist. _____time _____

avg. HR_____avg. power _____

zone 1_____2_____3_____4_____5_____

notes _____

_____

_____

_____

_____

_____

_____

_____

_____

_____

nutrition _____

_____

_____

_____

THURSDAY ____ / ____ / ____

▪ sleep ▪ fatigue ▪ stress ▪ soreness

resting heart rate_____ weight _____

WORKOUT 1 S B R O _____

planned workout_____

_____

route _____dist. _____time _____

avg. HR_____avg. power _____

zone 1_____2_____3_____4_____5_____

WORKOUT 2 S B R O _____

planned workout_____

_____

route _____dist. _____time _____

avg. HR_____avg. power _____

zone 1_____2_____3_____4_____5_____

notes _____

_____

_____

_____

_____

_____

_____

_____

_____

nutrition _____

_____

FRIDAY _____ / ____ / _____

░ sleep ░ fatigue ░ stress ░ soreness

resting heart rate _____ weight _____

WORKOUT 1 S B R 0 _____

planned workout _____

_____

_____

route _____ dist. _____ time _____

avg. HR _____ avg. power _____

zone 1 ____ 2 ____ 3 ____ 4 ____ 5 ____

WORKOUT 2 S B R 0 _____

planned workout _____

_____

route _____ dist. _____ time _____

avg. HR _____ avg. power _____

zone 1 ____ 2 ____ 3 ____ 4 ____ 5 ____

notes _____

_____

_____

_____

_____

_____

_____

_____

_____

_____

nutrition _____

_____

_____

_____

SATURDAY _____ / ____ / _____

░ sleep ░ fatigue ░ stress ░ soreness

resting heart rate _____ weight _____

WORKOUT 1 S B R 0 _____

planned workout _____

_____

_____

route _____ dist. _____ time _____

avg. HR _____ avg. power _____

zone 1 ____ 2 ____ 3 ____ 4 ____ 5 ____

WORKOUT 2 S B R 0 _____

planned workout _____

_____

_____

route _____ dist. _____ time _____

avg. HR _____ avg. power _____

zone 1 ____ 2 ____ 3 ____ 4 ____ 5 ____

notes _____

_____

_____

_____

_____

_____

_____

_____

_____

_____

nutrition _____

_____

_____

_____

SUNDAY _____ / _____ / _____

☐ sleep ☐ fatigue ☐ stress ☐ soreness

resting heart rate_____ weight _____

WORKOUT 1 S B R O _____

planned workout_____

_____

_____

route _____ dist. _____ time _____

avg. HR _____ avg. power _____

zone 1_____ 2_____ 3_____ 4_____ 5_____

WORKOUT 2 S B R O _____

planned workout_____

_____

route _____ dist. _____ time _____

avg. HR _____ avg. power _____

zone 1_____ 2_____ 3_____ 4_____ 5_____

notes _____

_____

_____

_____

_____

_____

_____

_____

_____

_____

_____

nutrition _____

_____

_____

_____

WEEKLY SUMMARY

	time	distance	YTD time	YTD distance
swim				
bike				
run				
strength				
other				
total				

notes

_____

_____

_____

_____

_____

_____

_____

period: _____   planned hours: _____

MONDAY _____ / _____ / _____

▨ sleep ▨ fatigue ▨ stress ▨ soreness

resting heart rate_____ weight _____

WORKOUT 1 S B R O _____

planned workout_____

_____

route _____dist. _____time _____

avg. HR_____avg. power_____

zone 1_____ 2_____ 3_____ 4_____ 5_____

WORKOUT 2 S B R O _____

planned workout_____

_____

route _____dist. _____time _____

avg. HR_____avg. power_____

zone 1_____ 2_____ 3_____ 4_____ 5_____

notes _____

_____

_____

_____

_____

_____

_____

_____

_____

_____

nutrition _____

_____

_____

_____

TUESDAY _____ / _____ / _____

▨ sleep ▨ fatigue ▨ stress ▨ soreness

resting heart rate_____ weight _____

WORKOUT 1 S B R O _____

planned workout_____

_____

route _____dist. _____time _____

avg. HR_____avg. power_____

zone 1_____ 2_____ 3_____ 4_____ 5_____

WORKOUT 2 S B R O _____

planned workout_____

_____

route _____dist. _____time _____

avg. HR_____avg. power_____

zone 1_____ 2_____ 3_____ 4_____ 5_____

notes _____

_____

_____

_____

_____

_____

_____

_____

_____

nutrition _____

_____

week goals: ■ _____

■ _____

■ _____

WEDNESDAY ___/___/___

■ sleep ■ fatigue ■ stress ■ soreness

resting heart rate_____weight _____

WORKOUT 1 S B R O _____

planned workout_____

_____

route _____dist. _____time _____

avg. HR_____avg. power_____

zone 1_____2_____3_____4_____5_____

WORKOUT 2 S B R O _____

planned workout_____

_____

route _____dist. _____time _____

avg. HR_____avg. power_____

zone 1_____2_____3_____4_____5_____

notes _____

_____

_____

_____

_____

_____

_____

_____

_____

_____

nutrition _____

_____

_____

_____

THURSDAY ___/___/___

■ sleep ■ fatigue ■ stress ■ soreness

resting heart rate_____weight _____

WORKOUT 1 S B R O _____

planned workout_____

_____

route _____dist. _____time _____

avg. HR_____avg. power_____

zone 1_____2_____3_____4_____5_____

WORKOUT 2 S B R O _____

planned workout_____

_____

route _____dist. _____time _____

avg. HR_____avg. power_____

zone 1_____2_____3_____4_____5_____

notes _____

_____

_____

_____

_____

_____

_____

_____

_____

_____

nutrition _____

_____

_____

FRIDAY _____ / _____ / _____

■ sleep ■ fatigue ■ stress ■ soreness

resting heart rate_____ weight _____

WORKOUT 1 S B R O _____

planned workout _____

_____

_____

route _____ dist. _____ time _____

avg. HR _____ avg. power _____

zone 1 ____ 2 ____ 3 ____ 4 ____ 5 ____

WORKOUT 2 S B R O _____

planned workout _____

_____

route _____ dist. _____ time _____

avg. HR _____ avg. power _____

zone 1 ____ 2 ____ 3 ____ 4 ____ 5 ____

notes _____

_____

_____

_____

_____

_____

_____

_____

_____

_____

nutrition _____

_____

_____

SATURDAY _____ / _____ / _____

■ sleep ■ fatigue ■ stress ■ soreness

resting heart rate_____ weight _____

WORKOUT 1 S B R O _____

planned workout _____

_____

_____

route _____ dist. _____ time _____

avg. HR _____ avg. power _____

zone 1 ____ 2 ____ 3 ____ 4 ____ 5 ____

WORKOUT 2 S B R O _____

planned workout _____

_____

_____

route _____ dist. _____ time _____

avg. HR _____ avg. power _____

zone 1 ____ 2 ____ 3 ____ 4 ____ 5 ____

notes _____

_____

_____

_____

_____

_____

_____

_____

_____

_____

nutrition _____

_____

_____

SUNDAY _____ / _____ / _____

☐ sleep ☐ fatigue ☐ stress ☐ soreness

resting heart rate_____ weight _____

WORKOUT 1 S B R O _____

planned workout _____

_____

_____

route _____ dist. _____ time _____

avg. HR _____ avg. power _____

zone 1_____ 2_____ 3_____ 4_____ 5_____

WORKOUT 2 S B R O _____

planned workout _____

_____

route _____ dist. _____ time _____

avg. HR _____ avg. power _____

zone 1_____ 2_____ 3_____ 4_____ 5_____

notes _____

_____

_____

_____

_____

_____

_____

_____

_____

_____

_____

_____

_____

nutrition _____

_____

_____

_____

WEEKLY SUMMARY

	time	distance	YTD time	YTD distance
swim				
bike				
run				
strength				
other				
total				

notes

_____

_____

_____

_____

_____

_____

_____

_____

_____

period: _____   planned hours: _____

MONDAY _____ / _____ /

▨ sleep ▨ fatigue ▨ stress ▨ soreness

resting heart rate_____ weight _____

WORKOUT 1 S B R 0 _____

planned workout _____

_____

route _____ dist. _____ time _____

avg. HR _____ avg. power _____

zone 1_____ 2_____ 3_____ 4_____ 5_____

WORKOUT 2 S B R 0 _____

planned workout _____

_____

route _____ dist. _____ time _____

avg. HR _____ avg. power _____

zone 1_____ 2_____ 3_____ 4_____ 5_____

notes _____

_____

_____

_____

_____

_____

_____

_____

_____

_____

_____

nutrition _____

_____

_____

_____

TUESDAY _____ / _____ /

▨ sleep ▨ fatigue ▨ stress ▨ soreness

resting heart rate_____ weight _____

WORKOUT 1 S B R 0 _____

planned workout _____

_____

route _____ dist. _____ time _____

avg. HR _____ avg. power _____

zone 1_____ 2_____ 3_____ 4_____ 5_____

WORKOUT 2 S B R 0 _____

planned workout _____

_____

route _____ dist. _____ time _____

avg. HR _____ avg. power _____

zone 1_____ 2_____ 3_____ 4_____ 5_____

notes _____

_____

_____

_____

_____

_____

_____

_____

_____

_____

_____

nutrition _____

_____

_____

week goals: ▇ _____

▇ _____

▇ _____

WEDNESDAY _____ / _____ / _____

▇ sleep ▇ fatigue ▇ stress ▇ soreness

resting heart rate_____ weight _____

WORKOUT 1 S B R O _____

planned workout _____

_____

route _____ dist. _____ time _____

avg. HR _____ avg. power _____

zone 1_____ 2_____ 3_____ 4_____ 5_____

WORKOUT 2 S B R O _____

planned workout _____

_____

route _____ dist. _____ time _____

avg. HR _____ avg. power _____

zone 1_____ 2_____ 3_____ 4_____ 5_____

notes _____

_____

_____

_____

_____

_____

_____

_____

_____

_____

nutrition _____

_____

_____

_____

THURSDAY _____ / _____ / _____

▇ sleep ▇ fatigue ▇ stress ▇ soreness

resting heart rate_____ weight _____

WORKOUT 1 S B R O _____

planned workout _____

_____

route _____ dist. _____ time _____

avg. HR _____ avg. power _____

zone 1_____ 2_____ 3_____ 4_____ 5_____

WORKOUT 2 S B R O _____

planned workout _____

_____

route _____ dist. _____ time _____

avg. HR _____ avg. power _____

zone 1_____ 2_____ 3_____ 4_____ 5_____

notes _____

_____

_____

_____

_____

_____

_____

_____

_____

_____

nutrition _____

_____

_____

_____

FRIDAY _____ / ___ / _____

■ sleep ■ fatigue ■ stress ■ soreness

resting heart rate _____ weight _____

WORKOUT 1 S B R O _____

planned workout _____

_____

_____

route _____ dist. _____ time _____

avg. HR _____ avg. power _____

zone 1 _____ 2 _____ 3 _____ 4 _____ 5 _____

WORKOUT 2 S B R O _____

planned workout _____

_____

route _____ dist. _____ time _____

avg. HR _____ avg. power _____

zone 1 _____ 2 _____ 3 _____ 4 _____ 5 _____

notes _____

_____

_____

_____

_____

_____

_____

_____

_____

nutrition _____

_____

_____

_____

SATURDAY _____ / ___ / _____

■ sleep ■ fatigue ■ stress ■ soreness

resting heart rate _____ weight _____

WORKOUT 1 S B R O _____

planned workout _____

_____

_____

route _____ dist. _____ time _____

avg. HR _____ avg. power _____

zone 1 _____ 2 _____ 3 _____ 4 _____ 5 _____

WORKOUT 2 S B R O _____

planned workout _____

_____

_____

route _____ dist. _____ time _____

avg. HR _____ avg. power _____

zone 1 _____ 2 _____ 3 _____ 4 _____ 5 _____

notes _____

_____

_____

_____

_____

_____

_____

_____

_____

_____

nutrition _____

_____

_____

_____

SUNDAY ___ / ___ / ___

☐ sleep ☐ fatigue ☐ stress ☐ soreness

resting heart rate_____ weight _____

WORKOUT 1 S B R O _____

planned workout _____

_____

route_____dist._____time _____

avg. HR_____avg. power_____

zone 1____ 2____ 3____ 4____ 5____

WORKOUT 2 S B R O _____

planned workout _____

_____

route_____dist._____time _____

avg. HR_____avg. power_____

zone 1____ 2____ 3____ 4____ 5____

notes _____

nutrition _____

WEEKLY SUMMARY

	time	distance	YTD time	YTD distance
swim				
bike				
run				
strength				
other				
total				

notes

period: _____ planned hours: _____

MONDAY ___ / ___ / ___

▢ sleep ▢ fatigue ▢ stress ▢ soreness

resting heart rate_____ weight _____

WORKOUT 1 S B R O _____

planned workout _____

_____

route _____ dist. _____ time _____

avg. HR _____ avg. power _____

zone 1____ 2____ 3____ 4____ 5____

WORKOUT 2 S B R O _____

planned workout _____

_____

route _____ dist. _____ time _____

avg. HR _____ avg. power _____

zone 1____ 2____ 3____ 4____ 5____

notes _____

_____

_____

_____

_____

_____

_____

_____

_____

_____

_____

nutrition _____

_____

_____

_____

TUESDAY ___ / ___ / ___

▢ sleep ▢ fatigue ▢ stress ▢ soreness

resting heart rate_____ weight _____

WORKOUT 1 S B R O _____

planned workout _____

_____

route _____ dist. _____ time _____

avg. HR _____ avg. power _____

zone 1____ 2____ 3____ 4____ 5____

WORKOUT 2 S B R O _____

planned workout _____

_____

route _____ dist. _____ time _____

avg. HR _____ avg. power _____

zone 1____ 2____ 3____ 4____ 5____

notes _____

_____

_____

_____

_____

_____

_____

_____

_____

_____

nutrition _____

_____

_____

week goals: ▪ _____

▪ _____

▪ _____

WEDNESDAY ____ / ____ / ____

▪ sleep ▪ fatigue ▪ stress ▪ soreness

resting heart rate_____ weight _____

WORKOUT 1 S B R O _____

planned workout_____

_____

route _____ dist. _____ time _____

avg. HR_____ avg. power _____

zone 1_____ 2_____ 3_____ 4_____ 5_____

WORKOUT 2 S B R O _____

planned workout_____

_____

route _____ dist. _____ time _____

avg. HR_____ avg. power _____

zone 1_____ 2_____ 3_____ 4_____ 5_____

notes _____

_____

_____

_____

_____

_____

_____

_____

_____

nutrition _____

_____

_____

THURSDAY ____ / ____ / ____

▪ sleep ▪ fatigue ▪ stress ▪ soreness

resting heart rate_____ weight _____

WORKOUT 1 S B R O _____

planned workout_____

_____

route _____ dist. _____ time _____

avg. HR_____ avg. power _____

zone 1_____ 2_____ 3_____ 4_____ 5_____

WORKOUT 2 S B R O _____

planned workout_____

_____

route _____ dist. _____ time _____

avg. HR_____ avg. power _____

zone 1_____ 2_____ 3_____ 4_____ 5_____

notes _____

_____

_____

_____

_____

_____

_____

_____

_____

nutrition _____

_____

_____

FRIDAY ___ / ___ / ___

■ sleep ■ fatigue ■ stress ■ soreness

resting heart rate_____ weight _____

WORKOUT 1 S B R O _____

planned workout _____

_____

_____

route _____ dist. _____ time _____

avg. HR _____ avg. power _____

zone 1_____ 2_____ 3_____ 4_____ 5_____

WORKOUT 2 S B R O _____

planned workout _____

_____

route _____ dist. _____ time _____

avg. HR _____ avg. power _____

zone 1_____ 2_____ 3_____ 4_____ 5_____

notes _____

_____

_____

_____

_____

_____

_____

_____

_____

_____

_____

nutrition _____

_____

_____

_____

SATURDAY ___ / ___ / ___

■ sleep ■ fatigue ■ stress ■ soreness

resting heart rate_____ weight _____

WORKOUT 1 S B R O _____

planned workout _____

_____

_____

route _____ dist. _____ time _____

avg. HR _____ avg. power _____

zone 1_____ 2_____ 3_____ 4_____ 5_____

WORKOUT 2 S B R O _____

planned workout _____

_____

route _____ dist. _____ time _____

avg. HR _____ avg. power _____

zone 1_____ 2_____ 3_____ 4_____ 5_____

notes _____

_____

_____

_____

_____

_____

_____

_____

_____

_____

nutrition _____

_____

_____

_____

SUNDAY _____ / ___ / _____

☐ sleep ☐ fatigue ☐ stress ☐ soreness

resting heart rate_____ weight _____

WORKOUT 1 S B R O _____

planned workout_____

_____

_____

route _____dist. _____time _____

avg. HR_____avg. power_____

zone 1_____2_____ 3_____ 4_____ 5_____

WORKOUT 2 S B R O _____

planned workout_____

_____

route _____dist. _____time _____

avg. HR_____avg. power_____

zone 1_____2_____ 3_____ 4_____ 5_____

notes _____

_____

_____

_____

_____

_____

_____

_____

_____

_____

_____

_____

nutrition _____

_____

_____

WEEKLY SUMMARY

	time	distance	YTD time	YTD distance
swim				
bike				
run				
strength				
other				
total				

notes

_____

_____

_____

_____

_____

_____

_____

_____

period: _____   planned hours: _____

MONDAY _____ / _____ / _____

▨ sleep ▨ fatigue ▨ stress ▨ soreness

resting heart rate_____ weight _____

WORKOUT 1 S B R O _____

planned workout _____

_____

route _____ dist. _____ time _____

avg. HR _____ avg. power _____

zone 1____ 2____ 3____ 4____ 5____

WORKOUT 2 S B R O _____

planned workout _____

_____

route _____ dist. _____ time _____

avg. HR _____ avg. power _____

zone 1____ 2____ 3____ 4____ 5____

notes _____

_____

_____

_____

_____

_____

_____

_____

_____

nutrition _____

_____

_____

_____

TUESDAY _____ / _____ / _____

▨ sleep ▨ fatigue ▨ stress ▨ soreness

resting heart rate_____ weight _____

WORKOUT 1 S B R O _____

planned workout _____

_____

route _____ dist. _____ time _____

avg. HR _____ avg. power _____

zone 1____ 2____ 3____ 4____ 5____

WORKOUT 2 S B R O _____

planned workout _____

_____

route _____ dist. _____ time _____

avg. HR _____ avg. power _____

zone 1____ 2____ 3____ 4____ 5____

notes _____

_____

_____

_____

_____

_____

_____

_____

_____

nutrition _____

_____

_____

week goals: ▪ _____

▪ _____

▪ _____

WEDNESDAY ____ / ____ / ____

▪ sleep ▪ fatigue ▪ stress ▪ soreness

resting heart rate_____ weight _____

WORKOUT 1 S B R O _____

planned workout _____

_____

route _____dist. _____time _____

avg. HR_____avg. power_____

zone 1_____ 2_____ 3_____ 4_____ 5_____

WORKOUT 2 S B R O _____

planned workout _____

_____

route _____dist. _____time _____

avg. HR_____avg. power_____

zone 1_____ 2_____ 3_____ 4_____ 5_____

notes _____

_____

_____

_____

_____

_____

_____

_____

_____

nutrition _____

_____

_____

_____

THURSDAY ____ / ____ / ____

▪ sleep ▪ fatigue ▪ stress ▪ soreness

resting heart rate_____ weight _____

WORKOUT 1 S B R O _____

planned workout _____

_____

route _____dist. _____time _____

avg. HR_____avg. power_____

zone 1_____ 2_____ 3_____ 4_____ 5_____

WORKOUT 2 S B R O _____

planned workout _____

_____

route _____dist. _____time _____

avg. HR_____avg. power_____

zone 1_____ 2_____ 3_____ 4_____ 5_____

notes _____

_____

_____

_____

_____

_____

_____

_____

nutrition _____

_____

_____

_____

FRIDAY _____ / ____ / _____

■ sleep ■ fatigue ■ stress ■ soreness

resting heart rate_____ weight _____

WORKOUT 1 S B R O _____

planned workout _____

_____

_____

route _____ dist. _____ time _____

avg. HR _____ avg. power _____

zone 1____ 2____ 3____ 4____ 5____

WORKOUT 2 S B R O _____

planned workout _____

_____

route _____ dist. _____ time _____

avg. HR _____ avg. power _____

zone 1____ 2____ 3____ 4____ 5____

notes _____

_____

_____

_____

_____

_____

_____

_____

_____

_____

nutrition _____

_____

_____

_____

SATURDAY _____ / ____ / _____

■ sleep ■ fatigue ■ stress ■ soreness

resting heart rate_____ weight _____

WORKOUT 1 S B R O _____

planned workout _____

_____

_____

route _____ dist. _____ time _____

avg. HR _____ avg. power _____

zone 1____ 2____ 3____ 4____ 5____

WORKOUT 2 S B R O _____

planned workout _____

_____

_____

route _____ dist. _____ time _____

avg. HR _____ avg. power _____

zone 1____ 2____ 3____ 4____ 5____

notes _____

_____

_____

_____

_____

_____

_____

_____

_____

_____

nutrition _____

_____

_____

_____

SUNDAY ___ / ___ / ___

☐ sleep ☐ fatigue ☐ stress ☐ soreness

resting heart rate _____ weight _____

WORKOUT 1 S B R O _____

planned workout _____

_____

_____

route _____ dist. _____ time _____

avg. HR _____ avg. power _____

zone 1 ___ 2 ___ 3 ___ 4 ___ 5 ___

WORKOUT 2 S B R O _____

planned workout _____

_____

route _____ dist. _____ time _____

avg. HR _____ avg. power _____

zone 1 ___ 2 ___ 3 ___ 4 ___ 5 ___

notes _____

_____
_____
_____
_____
_____
_____
_____
_____
_____

nutrition _____

_____
_____

WEEKLY SUMMARY

	time	distance	YTD time	YTD distance
swim				
bike				
run				
strength				
other				
total				

notes

week beginning: _____

period: _____   planned hours: _____

MONDAY _____ / _____ / _____

☐ sleep ☐ fatigue ☐ stress ☐ soreness

resting heart rate _____ weight _____

WORKOUT 1 S B R O _____

planned workout _____

_____

route _____ dist. _____ time _____

avg. HR _____ avg. power _____

zone 1____ 2____ 3____ 4____ 5____

WORKOUT 2 S B R O _____

planned workout _____

_____

route _____ dist. _____ time _____

avg. HR _____ avg. power _____

zone 1____ 2____ 3____ 4____ 5____

notes _____
_____
_____
_____
_____
_____
_____
_____
_____
_____

nutrition _____
_____
_____
_____

TUESDAY _____ / _____ / _____

☐ sleep ☐ fatigue ☐ stress ☐ soreness

resting heart rate _____ weight _____

WORKOUT 1 S B R O _____

planned workout _____

_____

route _____ dist. _____ time _____

avg. HR _____ avg. power _____

zone 1____ 2____ 3____ 4____ 5____

WORKOUT 2 S B R O _____

planned workout _____

_____

route _____ dist. _____ time _____

avg. HR _____ avg. power _____

zone 1____ 2____ 3____ 4____ 5____

notes _____
_____
_____
_____
_____
_____
_____
_____
_____

nutrition _____
_____
_____

week goals: ▪ _____

▪ _____

▪ _____

WEDNESDAY ____ / ____ / ____

▪ sleep ▪ fatigue ▪ stress ▪ soreness

resting heart rate _____ weight _____

WORKOUT 1 S B R O _____

planned workout _____

_____

route _____ dist. _____ time _____

avg. HR _____ avg. power _____

zone 1_____ 2_____ 3_____ 4_____ 5_____

WORKOUT 2 S B R O _____

planned workout _____

_____

route _____ dist. _____ time _____

avg. HR _____ avg. power _____

zone 1_____ 2_____ 3_____ 4_____ 5_____

notes _____

_____

_____

_____

_____

_____

_____

_____

_____

nutrition _____

_____

_____

_____

THURSDAY ____ / ____ / ____

▪ sleep ▪ fatigue ▪ stress ▪ soreness

resting heart rate _____ weight _____

WORKOUT 1 S B R O _____

planned workout _____

_____

route _____ dist. _____ time _____

avg. HR _____ avg. power _____

zone 1_____ 2_____ 3_____ 4_____ 5_____

WORKOUT 2 S B R O _____

planned workout _____

_____

route _____ dist. _____ time _____

avg. HR _____ avg. power _____

zone 1_____ 2_____ 3_____ 4_____ 5_____

notes _____

_____

_____

_____

_____

_____

_____

_____

_____

nutrition _____

_____

_____

_____

FRIDAY ___ / ___ / ___

■ sleep ■ fatigue ■ stress ■ soreness

resting heart rate_____ weight _____

WORKOUT 1 S B R O _____

planned workout _____

_____

_____

route _____ dist. _____ time _____

avg. HR_____ avg. power _____

zone 1_____ 2_____ 3_____ 4_____ 5_____

WORKOUT 2 S B R O _____

planned workout _____

_____

route _____ dist. _____ time _____

avg. HR_____ avg. power _____

zone 1_____ 2_____ 3_____ 4_____ 5_____

notes _____

_____

_____

_____

_____

_____

_____

_____

_____

_____

_____

nutrition _____

_____

_____

_____

SATURDAY ___ / ___ / ___

■ sleep ■ fatigue ■ stress ■ soreness

resting heart rate_____ weight _____

WORKOUT 1 S B R O _____

planned workout _____

_____

_____

route _____ dist. _____ time _____

avg. HR_____ avg. power _____

zone 1_____ 2_____ 3_____ 4_____ 5_____

WORKOUT 2 S B R O _____

planned workout _____

_____

route _____ dist. _____ time _____

avg. HR_____ avg. power _____

zone 1_____ 2_____ 3_____ 4_____ 5_____

notes _____

_____

_____

_____

_____

_____

_____

_____

_____

_____

nutrition _____

_____

_____

_____

SUNDAY _____ / ____ / _____

▢ sleep ▢ fatigue ▢ stress ▢ soreness

resting heart rate_____ weight _____

WORKOUT 1 S B R O _____

planned workout_____

_____

_____

route _____dist. _____time _____

avg. HR_____avg. power _____

zone 1_____2_____3_____4_____5_____

WORKOUT 2 S B R O _____

planned workout_____

_____

route _____dist. _____time _____

avg. HR_____avg. power _____

zone 1_____2_____3_____4_____5_____

notes _____

_____

_____

_____

_____

_____

_____

_____

_____

_____

_____

nutrition _____

_____

_____

_____

WEEKLY SUMMARY

	time	distance	YTD time	YTD distance
swim				
bike				
run				
strength				
other				
total				

notes

_____

_____

_____

_____

_____

_____

_____

_____

period: _____   planned hours: _____

MONDAY _____ / _____ /

▪ sleep ▪ fatigue ▪ stress ▪ soreness

resting heart rate_____ weight _____

WORKOUT 1 S B R O _____

planned workout _____

_____

route _____dist. _____time _____

avg. HR_____avg. power _____

zone 1_____ 2_____ 3_____ 4_____ 5_____

WORKOUT 2 S B R O _____

planned workout _____

_____

route _____dist. _____time _____

avg. HR_____avg. power _____

zone 1_____ 2_____ 3_____ 4_____ 5_____

notes _____

_____

_____

_____

_____

_____

_____

_____

_____

_____

nutrition _____

_____

_____

_____

TUESDAY _____ / _____ /

▪ sleep ▪ fatigue ▪ stress ▪ soreness

resting heart rate_____ weight _____

WORKOUT 1 S B R O _____

planned workout _____

_____

route _____dist. _____time _____

avg. HR_____avg. power _____

zone 1_____ 2_____ 3_____ 4_____ 5_____

WORKOUT 2 S B R O _____

planned workout _____

_____

route _____dist. _____time _____

avg. HR_____avg. power _____

zone 1_____ 2_____ 3_____ 4_____ 5_____

notes _____

_____

_____

_____

_____

_____

_____

_____

nutrition _____

_____

_____

week goals: ▪ _____

▪ _____

▪ _____

WEDNESDAY ___ / ___ / ___

▪ sleep ▪ fatigue ▪ stress ▪ soreness

resting heart rate_____ weight _____

WORKOUT 1 S B R O _____

planned workout_____

_____

route _____dist. _____time _____

avg. HR_____avg. power_____

zone 1_____ 2_____ 3_____ 4_____ 5_____

WORKOUT 2 S B R O _____

planned workout_____

_____

route _____dist. _____time _____

avg. HR_____avg. power_____

zone 1_____ 2_____ 3_____ 4_____ 5_____

notes _____

_____

_____

_____

_____

_____

_____

_____

_____

_____

nutrition _____

_____

_____

_____

THURSDAY ___ / ___ / ___

▪ sleep ▪ fatigue ▪ stress ▪ soreness

resting heart rate_____ weight _____

WORKOUT 1 S B R O _____

planned workout_____

_____

route _____dist. _____time _____

avg. HR_____avg. power_____

zone 1_____ 2_____ 3_____ 4_____ 5_____

WORKOUT 2 S B R O _____

planned workout_____

_____

route _____dist. _____time _____

avg. HR_____avg. power_____

zone 1_____ 2_____ 3_____ 4_____ 5_____

notes _____

_____

_____

_____

_____

_____

_____

_____

_____

_____

nutrition _____

_____

_____

_____

FRIDAY _____ / ____ / _____

sleep ▓ fatigue ▓ stress ▓ soreness

resting heart rate _____ weight _____

WORKOUT 1 S B R O _____

planned workout _____

_____

_____

route _____ dist. _____ time _____

avg. HR _____ avg. power _____

zone 1 ____ 2 ____ 3 ____ 4 ____ 5 ____

WORKOUT 2 S B R O _____

planned workout _____

_____

route _____ dist. _____ time _____

avg. HR _____ avg. power _____

zone 1 ____ 2 ____ 3 ____ 4 ____ 5 ____

notes _____

_____

_____

_____

_____

_____

_____

_____

_____

_____

nutrition _____

_____

_____

SATURDAY _____ / ____ / _____

sleep ▓ fatigue ▓ stress ▓ soreness

resting heart rate _____ weight _____

WORKOUT 1 S B R O _____

planned workout _____

_____

_____

route _____ dist. _____ time _____

avg. HR _____ avg. power _____

zone 1 ____ 2 ____ 3 ____ 4 ____ 5 ____

WORKOUT 2 S B R O _____

planned workout _____

_____

_____

route _____ dist. _____ time _____

avg. HR _____ avg. power _____

zone 1 ____ 2 ____ 3 ____ 4 ____ 5 ____

notes _____

_____

_____

_____

_____

_____

_____

_____

_____

_____

_____

_____

nutrition _____

_____

_____

SUNDAY _____ / ___ / _____

☐ sleep ☐ fatigue ☐ stress ☐ soreness

resting heart rate_____ weight _____

WORKOUT 1 S B R O _____

planned workout _____

_____

_____

route _____ dist. _____ time _____

avg. HR _____ avg. power _____

zone 1_____ 2_____ 3_____ 4_____ 5_____

WORKOUT 2 S B R O _____

planned workout _____

_____

route _____ dist. _____ time _____

avg. HR _____ avg. power _____

zone 1_____ 2_____ 3_____ 4_____ 5_____

notes _____

_____

_____

_____

_____

_____

_____

_____

_____

_____

_____

_____

_____

nutrition _____

_____

_____

_____

WEEKLY SUMMARY

	time	distance	YTD time	YTD distance
swim				
bike				
run				
strength				
other				
total				

notes

_____

_____

_____

_____

_____

_____

_____

_____

period: _____   planned hours: _____

MONDAY _____ / _____ / _____

▨ sleep ▨ fatigue ▨ stress ▨ soreness

resting heart rate_____ weight _____

WORKOUT 1 S B R O _____

planned workout _____

_____

route _____ dist. _____ time _____

avg. HR _____ avg. power _____

zone 1____ 2____ 3____ 4____ 5____

WORKOUT 2 S B R O _____

planned workout _____

_____

route _____ dist. _____ time _____

avg. HR _____ avg. power _____

zone 1____ 2____ 3____ 4____ 5____

notes _____

_____

_____

_____

_____

_____

_____

_____

_____

_____

nutrition _____

_____

_____

TUESDAY _____ / _____ / _____

▨ sleep ▨ fatigue ▨ stress ▨ soreness

resting heart rate_____ weight _____

WORKOUT 1 S B R O _____

planned workout _____

_____

route _____ dist. _____ time _____

avg. HR _____ avg. power _____

zone 1____ 2____ 3____ 4____ 5____

WORKOUT 2 S B R O _____

planned workout _____

_____

route _____ dist. _____ time _____

avg. HR _____ avg. power _____

zone 1____ 2____ 3____ 4____ 5____

notes _____

_____

_____

_____

_____

_____

_____

_____

_____

_____

nutrition _____

_____

_____

week goals: ■ _____

■ _____

■ _____

WEDNESDAY ____ / ____ / ____

■ sleep ■ fatigue ■ stress ■ soreness

resting heart rate_____ weight _____

WORKOUT 1 S B R O _____

planned workout_____

_____

route _____ dist. _____ time _____

avg. HR_____ avg. power_____

zone 1_____ 2_____ 3_____ 4_____ 5_____

WORKOUT 2 S B R O _____

planned workout_____

_____

route _____ dist. _____ time _____

avg. HR_____ avg. power_____

zone 1_____ 2_____ 3_____ 4_____ 5_____

notes _____

_____
_____
_____
_____
_____
_____
_____
_____
_____
_____

nutrition _____

_____
_____
_____

THURSDAY ____ / ____ / ____

■ sleep ■ fatigue ■ stress ■ soreness

resting heart rate_____ weight _____

WORKOUT 1 S B R O _____

planned workout_____

_____

route _____ dist. _____ time _____

avg. HR_____ avg. power_____

zone 1_____ 2_____ 3_____ 4_____ 5_____

WORKOUT 2 S B R O _____

planned workout_____

_____

route _____ dist. _____ time _____

avg. HR_____ avg. power_____

zone 1_____ 2_____ 3_____ 4_____ 5_____

notes _____

_____
_____
_____
_____
_____
_____
_____

nutrition _____

_____
_____
_____

FRIDAY _____ / _____ / _____

■ sleep ■ fatigue ■ stress ■ soreness

resting heart rate_____ weight _____

WORKOUT 1 S B R O _____

planned workout _____

_____

_____

route _____ dist. _____ time _____

avg. HR _____ avg. power _____

zone 1____ 2____ 3____ 4____ 5____

WORKOUT 2 S B R O _____

planned workout _____

_____

route _____ dist. _____ time _____

avg. HR _____ avg. power _____

zone 1____ 2____ 3____ 4____ 5____

notes _____

_____

_____

_____

_____

_____

_____

_____

_____

_____

_____

nutrition _____

_____

_____

_____

SATURDAY _____ / _____ / _____

■ sleep ■ fatigue ■ stress ■ soreness

resting heart rate_____ weight _____

WORKOUT 1 S B R O _____

planned workout _____

_____

_____

route _____ dist. _____ time _____

avg. HR _____ avg. power _____

zone 1____ 2____ 3____ 4____ 5____

WORKOUT 2 S B R O _____

planned workout _____

_____

route _____ dist. _____ time _____

avg. HR _____ avg. power _____

zone 1____ 2____ 3____ 4____ 5____

notes _____

_____

_____

_____

_____

_____

_____

_____

_____

_____

_____

nutrition _____

_____

_____

_____

SUNDAY _____ / ___ / _____

☐ sleep ☐ fatigue ☐ stress ☐ soreness

resting heart rate_____ weight _____

WORKOUT 1 S B R O _____

planned workout_____

_____

_____

route _____ dist. _____ time _____

avg. HR _____ avg. power _____

zone 1_____ 2_____ 3_____ 4_____ 5_____

WORKOUT 2 S B R O _____

planned workout_____

_____

route _____ dist. _____ time _____

avg. HR _____ avg. power _____

zone 1_____ 2_____ 3_____ 4_____ 5_____

notes _____

_____

_____

_____

_____

_____

_____

_____

_____

_____

_____

_____

nutrition _____

_____

_____

WEEKLY SUMMARY

	time	distance	YTD time	YTD distance
swim				
bike				
run				
strength				
other				
total				

notes

_____

_____

_____

_____

_____

_____

_____

period: _____   planned hours: _____

MONDAY _____ / ___ / _____

■ sleep ■ fatigue ■ stress ■ soreness

resting heart rate_____ weight _____

WORKOUT 1 S B R O _____

planned workout _____

_____

route _____ dist. _____ time _____

avg. HR _____ avg. power _____

zone 1____ 2____ 3____ 4____ 5____

WORKOUT 2 S B R O _____

planned workout _____

_____

route _____ dist. _____ time _____

avg. HR _____ avg. power _____

zone 1____ 2____ 3____ 4____ 5____

notes _____

_____
_____
_____
_____
_____
_____
_____
_____
_____

nutrition _____

_____
_____
_____
_____

TUESDAY _____ / ___ / _____

■ sleep ■ fatigue ■ stress ■ soreness

resting heart rate_____ weight _____

WORKOUT 1 S B R O _____

planned workout _____

_____

route _____ dist. _____ time _____

avg. HR _____ avg. power _____

zone 1____ 2____ 3____ 4____ 5____

WORKOUT 2 S B R O _____

planned workout _____

_____

route _____ dist. _____ time _____

avg. HR _____ avg. power _____

zone 1____ 2____ 3____ 4____ 5____

notes _____

_____
_____
_____
_____
_____
_____
_____
_____
_____

nutrition _____

_____
_____
_____

week goals: ◾ _____

◾ _____

◾ _____

WEDNESDAY _____ / _____ / _____

◾ sleep ◾ fatigue ◾ stress ◾ soreness

resting heart rate_____ weight _____

WORKOUT 1 S B R O _____

planned workout_____

_____

route _____ dist. _____ time _____

avg. HR_____ avg. power_____

zone 1_____ 2_____ 3_____ 4_____ 5_____

WORKOUT 2 S B R O _____

planned workout_____

_____

route _____ dist. _____ time _____

avg. HR_____ avg. power_____

zone 1_____ 2_____ 3_____ 4_____ 5_____

notes _____

_____

_____

_____

_____

_____

_____

_____

_____

_____

_____

nutrition _____

_____

_____

_____

THURSDAY _____ / _____ / _____

◾ sleep ◾ fatigue ◾ stress ◾ soreness

resting heart rate_____ weight _____

WORKOUT 1 S B R O _____

planned workout_____

_____

route _____ dist. _____ time _____

avg. HR_____ avg. power_____

zone 1_____ 2_____ 3_____ 4_____ 5_____

WORKOUT 2 S B R O _____

planned workout_____

_____

route _____ dist. _____ time _____

avg. HR_____ avg. power_____

zone 1_____ 2_____ 3_____ 4_____ 5_____

notes _____

_____

_____

_____

_____

_____

_____

_____

_____

_____

nutrition _____

_____

_____

FRIDAY _____ / _____ / _____

sleep ▨ fatigue ▨ stress ▨ soreness

resting heart rate _____ weight _____

WORKOUT 1 S B R O _____

planned workout _____

_____

_____

route _____ dist. _____ time _____

avg. HR _____ avg. power _____

zone 1 _____ 2 _____ 3 _____ 4 _____ 5 _____

WORKOUT 2 S B R O _____

planned workout _____

_____

route _____ dist. _____ time _____

avg. HR _____ avg. power _____

zone 1 _____ 2 _____ 3 _____ 4 _____ 5 _____

notes _____

_____

_____

_____

_____

_____

_____

_____

_____

_____

_____

nutrition _____

_____

_____

_____

SATURDAY _____ / _____ / _____

sleep ▨ fatigue ▨ stress ▨ soreness

resting heart rate _____ weight _____

WORKOUT 1 S B R O _____

planned workout _____

_____

_____

route _____ dist. _____ time _____

avg. HR _____ avg. power _____

zone 1 _____ 2 _____ 3 _____ 4 _____ 5 _____

WORKOUT 2 S B R O _____

planned workout _____

_____

route _____ dist. _____ time _____

avg. HR _____ avg. power _____

zone 1 _____ 2 _____ 3 _____ 4 _____ 5 _____

notes _____

_____

_____

_____

_____

_____

_____

_____

_____

_____

_____

nutrition _____

_____

_____

_____

SUNDAY ____ / ____ / ____

☐ sleep ☐ fatigue ☐ stress ☐ soreness

resting heart rate_____ weight _____

WORKOUT 1 S B R O _____

planned workout_____

_____

_____

route _____ dist. _____ time _____

avg. HR _____ avg. power _____

zone 1____ 2____ 3____ 4____ 5____

WORKOUT 2 S B R O _____

planned workout_____

_____

route _____ dist. _____ time _____

avg. HR _____ avg. power _____

zone 1____ 2____ 3____ 4____ 5____

notes _____

_____

_____

_____

_____

_____

_____

_____

_____

_____

_____

nutrition _____

_____

_____

_____

WEEKLY SUMMARY

	time	distance	YTD time	YTD distance
swim				
bike				
run				
strength				
other				
total				

notes

_____

_____

_____

_____

_____

_____

_____

_____

week beginning: _____

period: _____   planned hours: _____

MONDAY _____ / ____ / _____

▢ sleep ▢ fatigue ▢ stress ▢ soreness

resting heart rate_____ weight _____

WORKOUT 1 S B R O _____

planned workout_____

_____

route _____dist. _____time _____

avg. HR_____avg. power_____

zone 1_____ 2_____ 3_____ 4_____ 5_____

WORKOUT 2 S B R O _____

planned workout_____

_____

route _____dist. _____time _____

avg. HR_____avg. power_____

zone 1_____ 2_____ 3_____ 4_____ 5_____

notes _____

_____

_____

_____

_____

_____

_____

_____

_____

_____

nutrition _____

_____

_____

_____

TUESDAY _____ / ____ / _____

▢ sleep ▢ fatigue ▢ stress ▢ soreness

resting heart rate_____ weight _____

WORKOUT 1 S B R O _____

planned workout_____

_____

route _____dist. _____time _____

avg. HR_____avg. power_____

zone 1_____ 2_____ 3_____ 4_____ 5_____

WORKOUT 2 S B R O _____

planned workout_____

_____

route _____dist. _____time _____

avg. HR_____avg. power_____

zone 1_____ 2_____ 3_____ 4_____ 5_____

notes _____

_____

_____

_____

_____

_____

_____

_____

_____

nutrition _____

_____

week goals: ▪ _____

▪ _____

▪ _____

WEDNESDAY ____ / ____ / ____

▪ sleep ▪ fatigue ▪ stress ▪ soreness

resting heart rate_____ weight _____

WORKOUT 1 S B R O _____

planned workout _____

_____

route _____ dist. _____ time _____

avg. HR _____ avg. power _____

zone 1____ 2____ 3____ 4____ 5____

WORKOUT 2 S B R O _____

planned workout _____

_____

route _____ dist. _____ time _____

avg. HR _____ avg. power _____

zone 1____ 2____ 3____ 4____ 5____

notes _____

_____

_____

_____

_____

_____

_____

_____

_____

nutrition _____

_____

_____

_____

THURSDAY ____ / ____ / ____

▪ sleep ▪ fatigue ▪ stress ▪ soreness

resting heart rate_____ weight _____

WORKOUT 1 S B R O _____

planned workout _____

_____

route _____ dist. _____ time _____

avg. HR _____ avg. power _____

zone 1____ 2____ 3____ 4____ 5____

WORKOUT 2 S B R O _____

planned workout _____

_____

route _____ dist. _____ time _____

avg. HR _____ avg. power _____

zone 1____ 2____ 3____ 4____ 5____

notes _____

_____

_____

_____

_____

_____

_____

_____

_____

_____

_____

nutrition _____

_____

_____

FRIDAY _____ / _____ / _____

☐ sleep ☐ fatigue ☐ stress ☐ soreness

resting heart rate_____ weight _____

WORKOUT 1 S B R O _____

planned workout _____

_____

_____

route _____ dist. _____ time _____

avg. HR_____ avg. power_____

zone 1_____ 2_____ 3_____ 4_____ 5_____

WORKOUT 2 S B R O _____

planned workout _____

_____

route _____ dist. _____ time _____

avg. HR_____ avg. power_____

zone 1_____ 2_____ 3_____ 4_____ 5_____

notes _____

_____

_____

_____

_____

_____

_____

_____

_____

_____

_____

nutrition _____

_____

_____

_____

SATURDAY _____ / _____ / _____

☐ sleep ☐ fatigue ☐ stress ☐ soreness

resting heart rate_____ weight _____

WORKOUT 1 S B R O _____

planned workout _____

_____

_____

route _____ dist. _____ time _____

avg. HR_____ avg. power_____

zone 1_____ 2_____ 3_____ 4_____ 5_____

WORKOUT 2 S B R O _____

planned workout _____

_____

_____

route _____ dist. _____ time _____

avg. HR_____ avg. power_____

zone 1_____ 2_____ 3_____ 4_____ 5_____

notes _____

_____

_____

_____

_____

_____

_____

_____

_____

_____

nutrition _____

_____

_____

_____

SUNDAY _____ / ___ / _____

☐ sleep ☐ fatigue ☐ stress ☐ soreness

resting heart rate_____ weight _____

WORKOUT 1 S B R O _____

planned workout_____

_____

_____

route _____ dist. _____ time _____

avg. HR_____ avg. power _____

zone 1_____ 2_____ 3_____ 4_____ 5_____

WORKOUT 2 S B R O _____

planned workout_____

_____

route _____ dist. _____ time _____

avg. HR_____ avg. power _____

zone 1_____ 2_____ 3_____ 4_____ 5_____

notes _____

_____

_____

_____

_____

_____

_____

_____

_____

_____

_____

_____

nutrition _____

_____

_____

WEEKLY SUMMARY

	time	distance	YTD time	YTD distance
swim				
bike				
run				
strength				
other				
total				

notes

_____

_____

_____

_____

_____

_____

_____

_____

period: _____   planned hours: _____

MONDAY _____ / ____ / _____

▨ sleep ▨ fatigue ▨ stress ▨ soreness

resting heart rate_____ weight _____

WORKOUT 1 S B R O _____

planned workout_____

_____

route _____dist. _____time _____

avg. HR_____avg. power_____

zone 1_____2_____3_____4_____5_____

WORKOUT 2 S B R O _____

planned workout_____

_____

route _____dist. _____time _____

avg. HR_____avg. power_____

zone 1_____2_____3_____4_____5_____

notes _____

_____

_____

_____

_____

_____

_____

_____

_____

_____

_____

nutrition _____

_____

_____

_____

TUESDAY _____ / ____ / _____

▨ sleep ▨ fatigue ▨ stress ▨ soreness

resting heart rate_____ weight _____

WORKOUT 1 S B R O _____

planned workout_____

_____

route _____dist. _____time _____

avg. HR_____avg. power_____

zone 1_____2_____3_____4_____5_____

WORKOUT 2 S B R O _____

planned workout_____

_____

route _____dist. _____time _____

avg. HR_____avg. power_____

zone 1_____2_____3_____4_____5_____

notes _____

_____

_____

_____

_____

_____

_____

_____

_____

_____

nutrition _____

_____

_____

week goals: ▪ _____

▪ _____

▪ _____

WEDNESDAY ____ / ____ / ____

▪ sleep ▪ fatigue ▪ stress ▪ soreness

resting heart rate_____ weight _____

WORKOUT 1 S B R O _____

planned workout_____

_____

route _____dist. _____time _____

avg. HR_____avg. power_____

zone 1_____ 2_____ 3_____ 4_____ 5_____

WORKOUT 2 S B R O _____

planned workout_____

_____

route _____dist. _____time _____

avg. HR_____avg. power_____

zone 1_____ 2_____ 3_____ 4_____ 5_____

notes _____

_____

_____

_____

_____

_____

_____

_____

_____

_____

nutrition _____

_____

_____

_____

THURSDAY ____ / ____ / ____

▪ sleep ▪ fatigue ▪ stress ▪ soreness

resting heart rate_____ weight _____

WORKOUT 1 S B R O _____

planned workout_____

_____

route _____dist. _____time _____

avg. HR_____avg. power_____

zone 1_____ 2_____ 3_____ 4_____ 5_____

WORKOUT 2 S B R O _____

planned workout_____

_____

route _____dist. _____time _____

avg. HR_____avg. power_____

zone 1_____ 2_____ 3_____ 4_____ 5_____

notes _____

_____

_____

_____

_____

_____

_____

_____

_____

_____

nutrition _____

_____

_____

_____

FRIDAY ___/___/___

■ sleep ■ fatigue ■ stress ■ soreness

resting heart rate_____ weight _____

WORKOUT 1 S B R O _____

planned workout_____

_____

_____

route _____ dist. _____ time _____

avg. HR _____ avg. power _____

zone 1____ 2____ 3____ 4____ 5____

WORKOUT 2 S B R O _____

planned workout_____

_____

route _____ dist. _____ time _____

avg. HR _____ avg. power _____

zone 1____ 2____ 3____ 4____ 5____

notes _____

_____
_____
_____
_____
_____
_____
_____
_____
_____
_____

nutrition _____

_____
_____
_____

SATURDAY ___/___/___

■ sleep ■ fatigue ■ stress ■ soreness

resting heart rate_____ weight _____

WORKOUT 1 S B R O _____

planned workout_____

_____

_____

route _____ dist. _____ time _____

avg. HR _____ avg. power _____

zone 1____ 2____ 3____ 4____ 5____

WORKOUT 2 S B R O _____

planned workout_____

_____

route _____ dist. _____ time _____

avg. HR _____ avg. power _____

zone 1____ 2____ 3____ 4____ 5____

notes _____

_____
_____
_____
_____
_____
_____
_____
_____
_____

nutrition _____

_____
_____

SUNDAY ___ / ___ / ___

☐ sleep ☐ fatigue ☐ stress ☐ soreness

resting heart rate_____ weight _____

WORKOUT 1 S B R O _____

planned workout _____

_____

_____

route _____ dist. _____ time _____

avg. HR _____ avg. power _____

zone 1____ 2____ 3____ 4____ 5____

WORKOUT 2 S B R O _____

planned workout _____

_____

route _____ dist. _____ time _____

avg. HR _____ avg. power _____

zone 1____ 2____ 3____ 4____ 5____

notes _____

_____

_____

_____

_____

_____

_____

_____

_____

_____

_____

nutrition _____

_____

_____

_____

WEEKLY SUMMARY

	time	distance	YTD time	YTD distance
swim				
bike				
run				
strength				
other				
total				

notes

_____

_____

_____

_____

_____

_____

_____

DIARY PAGES

RACE _____ / / / _____ distance _____

location_____ time_____ placement overall_____ AG_____

	time	distance	pace	place
swim				
bike				
run				
transition 1				
transition 2				

nutrition pre-race_____

nutrition during race_____

avg. heart rate_____ max heart rate_____ avg. power_____

notes _____

_____

_____

RACE _____ / / / _____ distance _____

location_____ time_____ placement overall_____ AG_____

	time	distance	pace	place
swim				
bike				
run				
transition 1				
transition 2				

nutrition pre-race_____

nutrition during race_____

avg. heart rate_____ max heart rate_____ avg. power_____

notes _____

_____

_____

RACE _____ / / / _____ distance _____

location_____time_____ placement overall_____AG_____

	time	distance	pace	place
swim				
bike				
run				
transition 1				
transition 2				

nutrition pre-race_____

nutrition during race_____

avg. heart rate_____max heart rate_____avg. power_____

notes _____

_____

_____

RACE _____ / / / _____ distance _____

location_____time_____ placement overall_____AG_____

	time	distance	pace	place
swim				
bike				
run				
transition 1				
transition 2				

nutrition pre-race_____

nutrition during race_____

avg. heart rate_____max heart rate_____avg. power_____

notes _____

_____

_____

RACE _____ / / / _____ distance _____

location_____ time_____ placement overall_____ AG_____

	time	distance	pace	place
swim				
bike				
run				
transition 1				
transition 2				

nutrition pre-race_____

nutrition during race_____

avg. heart rate_____ max heart rate_____ avg. power_____

notes _____
_____
_____

RACE _____ / / / _____ distance _____

location_____ time_____ placement overall_____ AG_____

	time	distance	pace	place
swim				
bike				
run				
transition 1				
transition 2				

nutrition pre-race_____

nutrition during race_____

avg. heart rate_____ max heart rate_____ avg. power_____

notes _____
_____
_____

RACE _____ / / / distance _____
location_____ time_____ placement overall_____ AG_____

	time	distance	pace	place
swim				
bike				
run				
transition 1				
transition 2				

nutrition pre-race_____
nutrition during race_____
avg. heart rate_____ max heart rate_____ avg. power_____

notes _____
_____
_____

RACE _____ / / / distance _____
location_____ time_____ placement overall_____ AG_____

	time	distance	pace	place
swim				
bike				
run				
transition 1				
transition 2				

nutrition pre-race_____
nutrition during race_____
avg. heart rate_____ max heart rate_____ avg. power_____

notes _____
_____
_____

RACE _____ / / / _____ distance _____

location_____ time_____ placement overall_____ AG_____

	time	distance	pace	place
swim				
bike				
run				
transition 1				
transition 2				

nutrition pre-race_____

nutrition during race_____

avg. heart rate_____ max heart rate_____ avg. power_____

notes _____
_____
_____

RACE _____ / / / _____ distance _____

location_____ time_____ placement overall_____ AG_____

	time	distance	pace	place
swim				
bike				
run				
transition 1				
transition 2				

nutrition pre-race_____

nutrition during race_____

avg. heart rate_____ max heart rate_____ avg. power_____

notes _____
_____
_____

RACE _____ / / / _____ distance _____

location_____time_____ placement overall_____AG_____

	time	distance	pace	place
swim				
bike				
run				
transition 1				
transition 2				

nutrition pre-race_____

nutrition during race_____

avg. heart rate_____max heart rate_____avg. power_____

notes _____

_____

_____

RACE _____ / / / _____ distance _____

location_____time_____ placement overall_____AG_____

	time	distance	pace	place
swim				
bike				
run				
transition 1				
transition 2				

nutrition pre-race_____

nutrition during race_____

avg. heart rate_____max heart rate_____avg. power_____

notes _____

_____

_____

test results

DATE _____ / _____ / _____

test type _____

heart rate at AT_____

power at AT _____

	heart rate	power
zone 1	_____	_____
zone 2	_____	_____
zone 3	_____	_____
zone 4	_____	_____
zone 5a	_____	_____
zone 5b	_____	_____
zone 5c	_____	_____

VO_2max _____% body fat _____

notes _____

_____

_____

DATE _____ / _____ / _____

test type _____

heart rate at AT_____

power at AT _____

	heart rate	power
zone 1	_____	_____
zone 2	_____	_____
zone 3	_____	_____
zone 4	_____	_____
zone 5a	_____	_____
zone 5b	_____	_____
zone 5c	_____	_____

VO_2max _____% body fat _____

notes _____

_____

_____

DATE _____ / _____ / _____

test type _____

heart rate at AT_____

power at AT _____

	heart rate	power
zone 1	_____	_____
zone 2	_____	_____
zone 3	_____	_____
zone 4	_____	_____
zone 5a	_____	_____
zone 5b	_____	_____
zone 5c	_____	_____

VO_2max _____% body fat _____

notes _____

_____

_____

DATE _____ / _____ / _____

test type _____

heart rate at AT_____

power at AT _____

	heart rate	power
zone 1	_____	_____
zone 2	_____	_____
zone 3	_____	_____
zone 4	_____	_____
zone 5a	_____	_____
zone 5b	_____	_____
zone 5c	_____	_____

VO_2max _____% body fat _____

notes _____

_____

_____

DATE _____ / _____ / _____

test type _____

heart rate at AT_____

power at AT _____

	heart rate	power
zone 1		
zone 2		
zone 3		
zone 4		
zone 5a		
zone 5b		
zone 5c		

VO_2max _____% body fat _____

notes _____

_____

_____

DATE _____ / _____ / _____

test type _____

heart rate at AT_____

power at AT _____

	heart rate	power
zone 1		
zone 2		
zone 3		
zone 4		
zone 5a		
zone 5b		
zone 5c		

VO_2max _____% body fat _____

notes _____

_____

_____

DATE _____ / _____ / _____

test type _____

heart rate at AT_____

power at AT _____

	heart rate	power
zone 1		
zone 2		
zone 3		
zone 4		
zone 5a		
zone 5b		
zone 5c		

VO_2max _____% body fat _____

notes _____

_____

_____

DATE _____ / _____ / _____

test type _____

heart rate at AT_____

power at AT _____

	heart rate	power
zone 1		
zone 2		
zone 3		
zone 4		
zone 5a		
zone 5b		
zone 5c		

VO_2max _____% body fat _____

notes _____

_____

_____

When training information is graphed, trends are more easily seen. The grids provided on the next few pages could display weekly training hours or distances by sport; the longest weekly workout; the volume of weekly, race-specific intensity training (a good predictor of performance); or daily heart rates, either waking, recovery, or post-workout. You can probably come up with other creative ways to use this section. See page 17 for more ideas on how to use the following grids.

month

month

month

month

month

month

month

month

month

month

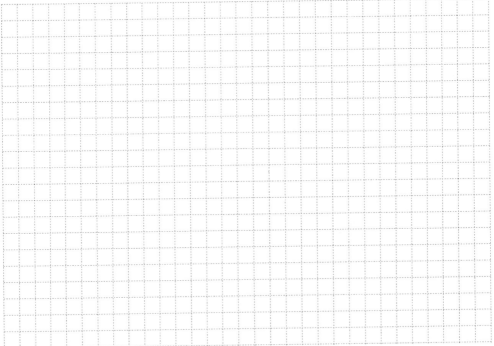

month

month

TRAINING GRIDS

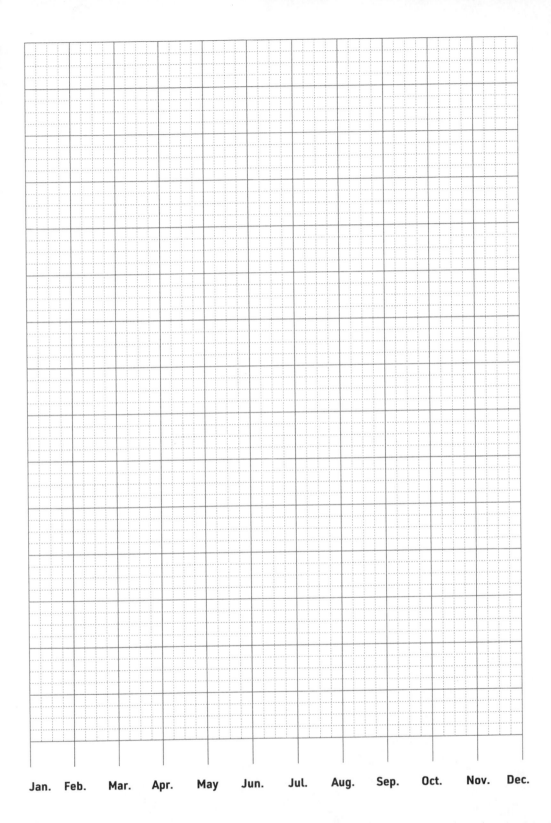

Jan.   Feb.   Mar.   Apr.   May   Jun.   Jul.   Aug.   Sep.   Oct.   Nov.   Dec.

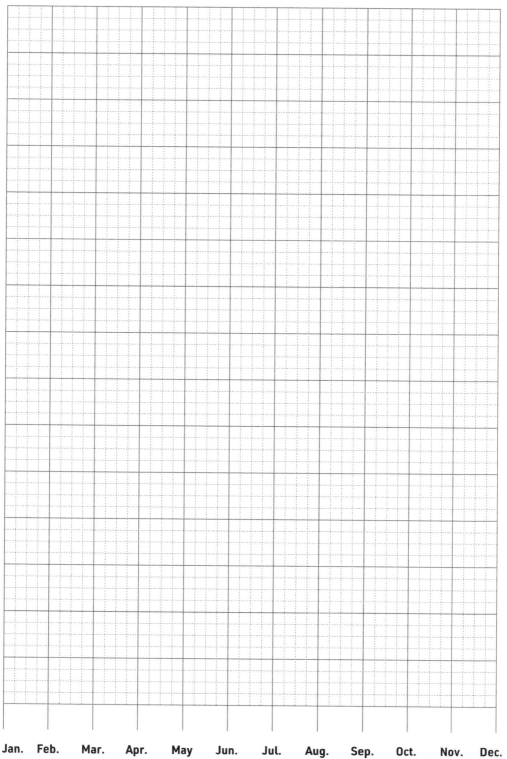

Jan. Feb. Mar. Apr. May Jun. Jul. Aug. Sep. Oct. Nov. Dec.

ROAD BIKE

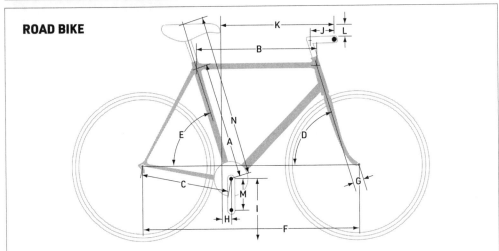

A. Seat tube length

B. Top tube length

C. Chainstay length

D. Head angle

E. Seat angle

F. Wheelbase

G. Fork offset

H. Seat setback

I. Bottom bracket height

J. Stem length

K. Reach

L. Seat-to-handlebar drop

M. Crank length

N. Seat height

Rear wheel spacing

Head tube diameter

Headset stack height

Seat tube diameter

Serial number

Date of purchase

■ *Seat height is measured from the center of the bottom bracket to the top of the saddle. The distance from the rails to the top of the saddle is not the same for all seats, so if you change saddles, this dimension may change.*

■ *Reach is measured from the nose of the saddle to the center of the bars. If you change saddles, remember that you may sit in a different position on the new saddle, and that may affect this dimension.*

■ *Crank length is measured from the center of the bottom bracket to the center of the pedal spindle.*

■ *Drop a weighted plumb line from the nose of the saddle to determine seat setback from the center of the bottom bracket.*

equipment changes

date	component	what was changed

MOUNTAIN BIKE

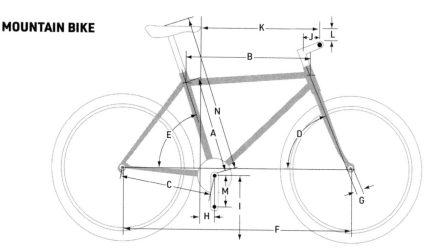

A. Seat tube length

B. Top tube length

C. Chainstay length

D. Head angle

E. Seat angle

F. Wheelbase

G. Fork offset

H. Seat setback

I. Bottom bracket height

J. Stem length

K. Reach

L. Seat-to-handlebar drop

M. Crank length

N. Seat height

Rear wheel spacing

Head tube diameter

Headset stack height

Seat tube diameter

Serial number

Date of purchase

■ *Seat height is measured from the center of the bottom bracket to the top of the saddle. The distance from the rails to the top of the saddle is not the same for all seats, so if you change saddles, this dimension may change.*

■ *Reach is measured from the nose of the saddle to the center of the bars. If you change saddles, remember that you may sit in a different position on the new saddle, and that may affect this dimension.*

■ *Crank length is measured from the center of the bottom bracket to the center of the pedal spindle.*

■ *Drop a weighted plumb line from the nose of the saddle to determine seat setback from the center of the bottom bracket.*

equipment changes		
date	component	what was changed

routes
and best times

route	date	time

season results

date	race	distance	place	comments

race-day checklist

To reduce pre-race stress and the possibility of forgetting an important item of clothing or equipment, use this checklist before leaving the house for your race. Better yet, use it the night before. You may not need everything, but you'll be sure to have it if the need arises.

- swim suit
- goggles
- wetsuit
- swim cap
- bike
- socks
- bike shoes
- helmet
- sunglasses
- gloves
- water bottle
- water/energy drink
- food/energy bars

- running shoes
- jersey/singlet
- bike shorts
- sunscreen
- towel
- petroleum jelly
- pump
- tools
- lubricant
- spare cogs/wheels
- race number
- parking permit (if issued)
- safety pins